50 STEPS
TO THE BEST
VERSION OF
YOURSELF

BLOOMSBURY SPORT

Bloomsbury Publishing Plc

50 Bedford Square, London, WC1B 3DP, UK

29 Earlsfort Terrace, Dublin 2, Ireland

BLOOMSBURY, BLOOMSBURY SPORT and the Diana logo are trademarks of Bloomsbury Publishing Plc

First published in Great Britain 2021

Copyright © Anton Danyluk, 2021

Original photography by Jenna Bussey

Design by D.R. ink

Pattern imagery © Shutterstock/Amovitania

With special thanks to Lisa Hughes, Adrian Besley and Cici Shannon,
and Kate O'Shea, Felan Davidson and all the team at Bold Management

A catalogue record for this book is available from the British Library

Library of Congress Cataloguing-in-Publication data has been applied for
add where a UK originated single-ISBN edition for which we own US rights

ISBN: PB; 978-1-4729-8781-5; eBook: 978-1-4729-8780-8 / 978-1-4729-8779-2

2 4 6 8 10 9 7 5 3 1

Printed in China by RRD Asia Printing Solutions Limited

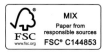

MIX
Paper from
responsible sources
FSC® C144853
www.fsc.org

To find out more about our authors and books visit www.bloomsbury.com and sign up for our newsletters

ANTON DANYLUK

50 STEPS TO THE BEST VERSION OF YOURSELF

BLOOMSBURY SPORT
LONDON • OXFORD • NEW YORK • NEW DELHI • SYDNEY

CONTENTS

INTRODUCTION

This book is about living your best possible life – and by best life I mean a healthy life that makes you feel happy and fulfilled. As well as my thoughts and advice, I've also devised a workout programme to help you kickstart (or restart) your journey to fitness, and I tell my story, including what it was like to become famous through a reality show like *Love Island*. We all have the potential to improve our lives, in terms not just of our health, but also our relationships, our work and the way we think about ourselves. My aim is to show you the simple steps you can take and pass on what I've learned.

You wouldn't think it to look at me today, but I was an overweight teenager – and being overweight made me miserable. Today I'm a qualified fitness and wellbeing expert, and gym owner. Of course, that change didn't happen overnight. It was the result of a series of small changes in what I did and how I thought – and they're all changes that you can make in your life too.

I'm interested in helping as many people as I can to become healthier and happier, and I always had a plan to raise my public profile enough so that I could make a difference. When World Merit asked me to be an ambassador for their UN-partnered Sustainable Development programme to promote good health and wellbeing, I felt that plan had come together!

Much of my time is now spent travelling up and down the country talking to young people. I try to communicate the benefits of being fit and healthy – and give them the confidence and motivation to eat well, exercise and look after themselves. It's the most rewarding thing I have ever done and if the message gets through to just one person, it will be worthwhile.

If you're thinking about where you are in your life and how to achieve your aspirations, I hope this book gives you some ideas and helps you find the motivation to change for the better. My philosophy is all about positivity and self-worth. If we believe in ourselves enough and have the determination to succeed, we can be whatever we want – we can not only reach for the stars, but touch them too.

Anton

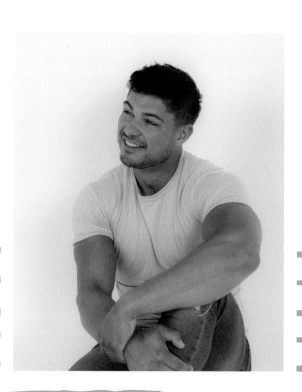

Positive mental health

Before you can get your body and, indeed, your life in good shape, you need to make sure that your mind is in good shape. The way to achieve that is by understanding who you are, being confident and motivated, and living in the moment.

1. Self-reflection

How well do you really know yourself? It's probably a lot less than you think. Our rush-around lives don't leave a lot a time to work out what we're doing, and how and why we're doing it. So maybe it's time to stop and say, 'Hi, me… Meet me.'

It's certainly not selfish or egotistical to spend a few moments assessing how you live your life. We all look in the mirror, what, 10 or even 20 times a day? We check our hair, make-up, clothes – sometimes pretty intensely. Most of us don't pay anything like that kind of attention to what we're thinking, planning and doing. Self-reflection is just about getting to know yourself better. It's becoming aware of your goals, your motivation, your relationships with other people and your happiness levels.

Getting to know yourself

Self-awareness is at the heart of living your best possible life because it reveals what you're capable of and what might get in the way of achieving your goals. Whether your focus is work, body image, friendships or romance, identifying your strengths, weaknesses, what you're proud of and what you hope to achieve in the future will help give you the confidence and drive to make improvements to your life. Basically, it can help you draw a road map to get where you want to go in the quickest and easiest way possible.

You shouldn't feel you have to meditate, lock yourself in a dark room or spend hours in thought. Self-reflection doesn't have to be an inventory of your innermost thoughts and can be achieved in just a few minutes. If you're the kind of person who won't otherwise get around to it (some quick self-reflection will tell you if you are!), maybe sitting down at a regular time every week will help you – and if you like taking notes, that's fine too. Your experiences and decisions affect the way you feel, so the important thing is that you make space in your life to check up on yourself.

Be firm but fair

You have to be prepared to ask yourself the tough questions. *What am I doing wrong? Am I the kind of person I want to be? Do I give in to temptation too easily?* You need to self-critical, but don't be judgemental or beat yourself up. Find the positives and use them. Build your confidence and remind yourself that you can make change happen. They can be small steps in your day-to-day life or long-term plans. Just be sure that you know they are achievable.

The self-reflection rules

▶ **Be honest with yourself.** We can all be too self-critical at times, so this means being honest about the positives as well as the negatives.

▶ **Challenge your assumptions.** Just because things have been a certain way in the past, it doesn't mean they have to be the same way in the future.

▶ **Deal with what you can control – not what you can't.** Sometimes it's not easy to work out which is which, but make the effort and then make sure you let go of what's beyond your control.

▶ **Remember your successes and achievements.** It's not boastful. As long as you're truthful, there's really nothing wrong with reminding yourself of these from time to time.

▶ **Focus on how change could improve your life.** Perhaps you need to work towards a few small changes or maybe it's one big, momentous change, but either way you owe it to yourself to give this some serious attention.

▶ **Revisit your conclusions and goals regularly.** This is important, because you will change over time and what you want from life may change as well, so check everything still lines up.

▶ **Like most things, self-reflection is a skill** you need to learn and practise, but the ability to think clearly about yourself is key to self-improvement.

2. Build your self-confidence

Belief in your own abilities is key to success. Self-confidence might not come naturally to you, but you can still develop a positive and adventurous attitude that can make positive things happen in every area of your life.

When I came out of *Love Island*, one of my first public engagements was giving a talk to over a thousand people at a grand hotel for a prestigious event. When I told people I was nervous about speaking at the event, they laughed, saying, 'You've just been on TV, parading yourself in front of millions of people!' That was true, but now I was out of my depth. Being the easy-going Anton was simple for me, but I was just a trainer and gym owner. Was I really the right person to inspire people to see the links between physical and mental health?

Everyone is shy sometimes

We are all capable of being confident — but that doesn't mean we can't sometimes feel shy, nervous and afraid of failure. It was a mixture of these that made me want to cancel that hotel event, but I had committed myself to speaking as part of my role as a World Merit Ambassador for the UN, and there was no way out. Looking out at all those people with their eyes locked on me, I was terrified and concerned I would make a complete fool of myself. *What if I opened my mouth and nothing came out? What if they laughed at me?* I had to dig deep to find the confidence to speak, but I was so pleased I did and it gave me a massive buzz – one of the greatest feelings of my life.

That's why it's so vital to build your self-confidence. It can have a massive effect on your life, enabling you to meet new people, try new experiences, and overcome obstacles and setbacks. It's a bit like growing wings. And we can all do it. If you think being introverted and shy prevents you, then look at Emma Watson, Lady Gaga, Zayn Malik or Lionel Messi – all who have overcome their natural shyness to succeed.

Confidence is a skill. You can train yourself to be confident just as you can learn to cook, knit or skateboard. Begin by acknowledging what you're capable of doing: relationships you've worked at, skills you have mastered and difficult situations you have managed. Only harsh self-criticism and fear of failing are stopping you from developing these attributes, so a promise to go easy on yourself and a vow to be adventurous can be the first steps to a fuller life.

Practice does makes perfect

Just like those other skills, a sense of self-confidence won't appear overnight. Try to stop concentrating on the obstacles preventing you from reaching your goals, and focus on the personal characteristics which will help you find a way round them. I spent ages rehearsing my speech in front of the mirror to make sure I got it right. I truly believe that with practice, determination and perhaps a little support you can achieve things you never thought possible – because it's true! When you find that positivity, project it. Stand straight, smile and look others in the eye, and you'll be amazed at the response – people like and respond to people who come across as confident.

Inside, of course, you might be quaking with fear. I certainly was during the sleepless night before that hotel speech. Overcoming those fears is the most difficult, but ultimately most rewarding, way of growing your self-confidence. Motivational speaker Jia Jiang suggests a rejection therapy that challenges people to deliberately seek out failure in their everyday lives. This may be a little extreme, but facing your fears – taking failure on the chin or enjoying the success – is part of the process. Feel the fear, and do it anyway!

Boosting your self-confidence

▶ Back yourself to succeed.

▶ Dress and groom to make yourself feel good.

▶ Acknowledge your strengths, challenge your insecurities.

▶ Prepare yourself properly for daunting meetings or endeavours.

▶ Take yourself out of your comfort zone on a regular basis.

▶ Accept mistakes and setbacks as part of growth.

3. Stay positive

Positivity is more than smiling through thick and thin and being constantly cheerful, it's making the mental effort to seek out opportunities for personal growth and actively looking to overcome the obstacles that stand in your way.

If you watch *Love Island,* you'll know it has its own language, with getting 'pied' – as in rejected or dumped by a love interest – the expression that is probably the most commonly used. And if there's one person associated with getting pied, it's yours truly! It wasn't pleasant getting rejected in front of millions of viewers and it definitely tested my powers of positivity.

I'm generally a positive person, but finding the positive side of everything isn't always easy. I don't want to sound arrogant, but being dumped by a girl was a situation I'd never really had to face before going on the programme and it did come as a shock – especially when it happened again and again! I went to my room thinking, 'WTF is going on here?' It would have been easy to feel angry or sorry for myself, but what would I have gained? I decided to laugh along at the situation and show people what I was really like.

Don't grin through gritted teeth

Having a positive attitude is not about grinning through disappointment and misfortune, but considering the opportunities, benefits and responses you can make to those situations. It's looking at life with a broad perspective rather than concentrating on single issues, and asking what can be done rather than believing it is all impossible. Research has shown that positivity has a number of health benefits, from resistance to colds and viruses to a healthier heart condition and, of course, being less prone to depression. Positive thinking can also lead to good fortune. It's not mysticism or superstition; you're just opening yourself up to opportunities, and most people react better to a smile and a can-do attitude. Although not everyone finds it easy to take a positive view of difficult situations, it's an approach anyone can train themselves to take.

Positivity training

▶ **Give yourself time.** Shocks and catastrophes happen, and sometimes you need a moment – or more – to process your thoughts, assess the situation and even to mourn.

▶ **Show self-compassion.** Console and encourage yourself as you would your best friend.

▶ **Try turning every negative into a positive:** *can* not can't, *will* not won't, *do* not don't.

▶ **Avoid negative influences.** If certain friends or social media sites upset you or make you feel negative, steer clear of them, either temporarily or permanently.

▶ **Retain your sense of humour.** Be prepared to laugh at yourself or your situation.

▶ **Focus on practical solutions.** Concentrate on solving the issue rather than worrying about it.

▶ **Always try to keep things in perspective.** This can be tricky, but if you can view an incident or feeling as 'small' in a 'larger' landscape, then you'll find it much easier to stay positive and move on.

4. Getting and staying motivated

Achieving your goals is all about motivation. Not just the initial get-up-and-go, but keeping up your commitment over time. If you can learn to negotiate the obstacles in your path and be inspired by the journey, you'll be well on the way.

Look at it this way. We're born motivated, right? We have the impulse to get out into the world: we learn to walk, speak, cross the road. And that impulse never goes away. We get dressed, go shopping… Hey, even reaching for the TV remote is a decision we make and act on. We just need to ramp up that inner motivation, channel it and direct it towards new challenges.

Set yourself up to win

You need a goal. It needs to be something you really want to achieve. Don't spread yourself too thin by trying to achieve a range of goals at the same time. Stick to one that you can focus on 100%. If it's a major undertaking, your first job is to break it down into small steps. Plot a first objective that you can reasonably expect to achieve in a short amount of time – days or weeks rather than months or years – and one you can definitely measure – don't smoke for *a week*, lose *four* pounds, run for *10 minutes* without stopping. Once you've ticked that off, move onto the next step. Create a positive cycle where success inspires you to achieve more and more.

Expect that your initial enthusiasm will eventually wane, so prepare yourself for days which you just have to get through. Your motivation will continue to ebb and flow, because of course it's going to be affected by external events and your own moods. Don't be put off too easily, though. Excuses are always easy to find. You don't have time? Make time. No matter who we are, we all have the same hours in our day. You're not progressing fast enough? Change your strategy and go

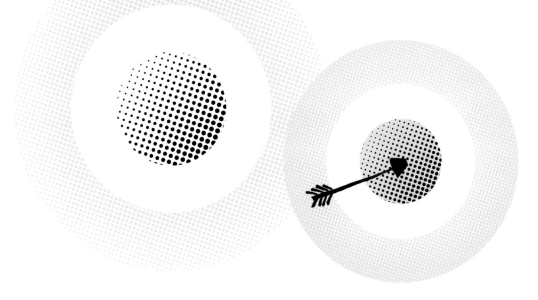

again. Remember what set you off on your goal in the first place. As long as your reasons outweigh the possible excuses, you can find the will to carry on.

It's all about you

Understand your personality and the obstacles it might present. When I was trying to lose weight, I knew I would find it difficult to go on a night out with my pals without eating and drinking. So I persuaded them to go hill walking the following day instead. There are other pitfalls as well as temptation. Could a lack of confidence or a desire to be perfect get in your way? If you lack determination, try getting a friend to join you, because you might find letting them down is more difficult than letting yourself down. Setting a goal won't turn you into a different person, so if you're going to stay motivated, you have to do it your own way.

You also need to be kind to yourself. Being your own harshest critic is as likely to demotivate you as spur you on. We're only human, and setbacks and mistakes are bound to happen. Acknowledge and take responsibility for failures, and avoid wallowing in frustration, self-pity or disappointment. Research has shown that people who show self-compassion are less likely to give up, and more inclined to set new goals and start over again. Don't think of it as going easy on yourself – it's about encouraging yourself to learn from your mistakes and become a stronger person.

5. Embrace opportunity

Opportunities are everywhere in life. Sometimes you need to work to make them happen, other times they open up when you weren't looking for them. But once you've found them, it's just a matter of determination, self-belief and bravery...

When I was offered the chance to go on *Love Island*, there were so many reasons for me to turn it down. I had no desire to be a 'reality show celebrity' and certainly wasn't looking for love. I'd be taking time out from running a successful business I had worked so long to build, and a prolonged absence might set it back. Plus the mere thought of being on the show scared me to death. It seemed such a big deal to bare myself (literally!) to millions of viewers, putting my personality, looks and behaviour up for public judgement. Then I signed up for it.

I had to. It promised excitement, fun and an incredible adventure into the unknown – an opportunity I knew would probably never come again. I relished the idea of being on one of the UK's most popular TV shows and although I reckoned I had as good a chance as anyone of winning – or being first out! – that was never on my mind. I was in it for two reasons: the experience of a lifetime and the opportunity to raise my profile in order to promote my kids' fitness programme.

There's a whole world out there

Recognising and grasping the opportunities the world presents is a key to living your best life. Sometimes you have to dig for them, earn them or make them; sometimes they offer themselves up; and occasionally you stumble over them. They're usually not flagged or lit up in neon, so you need to be alert to spot them. However, an open mind, a positive attitude and a willingness to embrace change is the best way to encounter a golden opportunity.

The future is yours to shape how you want. You certainly don't have to drag the past along with you. Unhappy schooldays, bad relationships, dismal jobs can all be bagged up and left in the bin. And your current life is never your only option. If you want to change it, you can. So many people find themselves doing things they never dreamed they would be capable of, they just needed to take one step.

Don't fear failure

The biggest obstacle to taking any opportunity is fear of failure. We might embarrass or humiliate ourselves, be mocked by others or find ourselves rejected. These were certainly all possible outcomes when I accepted the challenge to go on television. These fears can have a number of causes, varying from childhood experience to previous mistakes. They can result in us putting up our own obstacles, like drawn-out procrastination, an inability to make a final decision, a lack of confidence in our own abilities or a desire to only do things we can execute perfectly. Ultimately, you have a choice whether to scale these self-made fences or not, but there are strategies that can help.

How to make the change

▶ **Question your anxieties**. Are they real problems or ones you're creating?

▶ **Picture the future.** How will you overcome problems? What will success look like?

▶ **If you're always learning, you are never failing.**

▶ **Practise stepping out of your comfort zone.** What's the worst that can happen? It's usually not as bad as that.

▶ **Have a safety net.** A plan B you can fall back on can make you feel more secure

▶ **Just enjoy the ride!** Learn to accept the fear, adrenaline rush and stepping into the unknown as part of life's adventure.

6. Exercise is medicine

When my grandad died in 2015 it was the first time I'd ever coped with anything so tough. It hit my mother and me like a sledgehammer, but we reacted in different ways: my mother couldn't get out of bed and I couldn't get out of the gym.

Working out in the gym keeps me sane. It makes me feel better when I'm suffering from self-doubt, feeling angry, frustrated or upset. I don't do meditation (I'm not sure I can stay still for long enough!), but I understand the appeal because the focus and effort of exercise has that same effect of clearing the mind. It's impossible to even think for a second about your troubles when you're pushing through your third set of reps or gasping for breath on the last couple of ks of your run.

Trigger those endorphins

It's more than that. Everyone knows that exercise is great for your physical health, but there is also a scientifically proven link between physical exercise and positive mental health. It can lower stress, improve mood states and alleviate anxiety, and there is plenty of evidence that it might even prevent us falling into bouts of depression. The chemicals – including endorphins – which your body releases when you exercise in order to reduce your perception of pain also trigger a euphoric feeling, a flood of positive emotions sometimes called a 'runners' high'. While this may not last long, it can be enough to jolt you out of a fug or change your outlook on life.

It doesn't have to be a gym workout. You might prefer running, playing sport or even get enough benefit from a brisk walk. The important thing is that you push yourself enough to challenge your mind as well as your body. You won't regret it… I've never once left the gym saying I wish I hadn't done that.

'Emotion is created by motion'

The American life coach Tony Robbins is one of my heroes. His writing and podcasts on resetting your mind and mood have deeply influenced the way I try to help those I'm training. Robbins has one particular saying which especially resonates with me: 'Emotion is created by motion.' Just as how you feel physically affects how you feel emotionally, so the reverse is true. Although exercise is an obvious way of changing our physical state, even changing the way we move – jumping up and down, shaking out our body, even changing our posture – can help alter our mood.

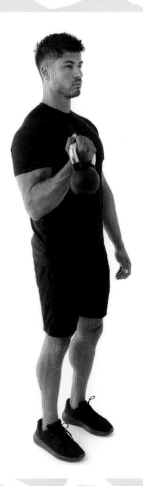

7. Body image

We can all find fault with the way we look. Some people are obsessed with spots, while others convince themselves they're carrying a bit of extra weight, but it's about time we gave ourselves a break and stopped worrying…

It would be great to live in Insta Land where everyone looks so gorgeous and healthy all the time, but it's a fake world, as much a fantasy as Neverland or Hogwarts. Celebs and influencers generally only ever post photos of themselves looking fabulous and many of those are retouched to give a perfect impression. Back on Earth, social media can be great for finding positive and even inspirational pics, but it's all too easy to compare yourself with others – and from there it's a short step to feeling inadequate or setting yourself unrealistic goals.

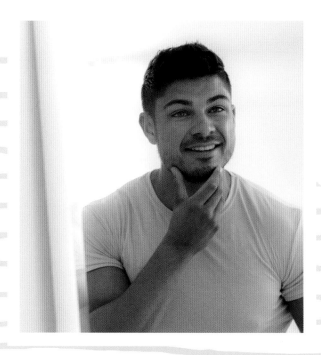

You are beautiful

That might seem odd coming from someone whose six-pack is often on display online. I'm proud of how I look and work hard at maintaining a toned body. After all, it's my job. No one wants a fitness trainer who looks out of shape. However, I've coached many people who look in the mirror and become despondent about what they see. Muscle dysmorphia – also called bigorexia – is a kind of reverse anorexia by which people see themselves as underbuilt and not buff enough, despite having highly developed muscles. It's increasingly common among gym-goers, which shows just how easy it is to get a distorted image of what you look like.

We really have become overcritical of our own bodies. It can be difficult, but you need to be straight with yourself. Recognise the things you like about your looks – it's not about being boastful, just be honest. Then think about what you don't like. Maybe you're not keen on the shape of your nose or the size of your feet, but work on accepting them. Beauty lies in the fact we are all unique, and we all have features – our eyes, our smile, our expressions, our hands or even the way we walk – that make us attractive. If you like what you see, so will others – guaranteed. Focus on being a better person: love yourself and practise confidence.

Don't be so judgemental

Yes, there are some things we may be able to change if we choose to, such as our hair style, our posture and our weight. It can be a complex psychological issue, but far too many people think their 'problem' is their weight. Perhaps carrying some excess fat can upset us or makes us determined to lose it, but the sooner you ditch the judgemental mindset, the sooner you can deal with any issues in a realistic way.

We are often bullied by our own brains which develop a warped perspective based on what we see around us. We need to fight back to develop a sensible relationship with our own body. Nearly all of us care about what we look like. That isn't a problem. It's thinking our body image defines who we are that's the issue. We have other attributes that are far more powerful, such as personalities and abilities, so build your self-worth and confidence around those. When you realise that an inner balance beats an outer balance every time, self-acceptance becomes so much easier.

8. Live in the moment

It's difficult to stop and appreciate life, there's too much going on. But if you can find a moment's clarity between work, worries, friends and commitments, I promise you it will be worth it.

One of my favourite moments on *Love Island* was when Craig David turned up to give an impromptu concert. I've been a massive Craig David fan for years and have gone out to Ibiza to see him perform almost every year. But this was different. On the show we were in a bubble; without phones, TVs or any other distractions. My appreciation of that gig surpassed anything I had seen and it was down to my ability to take in every detail. The emotion of the moment was enough to bring tears to my eyes – as many watching noticed!

Take your time

Modern life gets in the way of those moments. Everything seems to happen so fast and is blurred by our worries about how we look, what we said, what's going on somewhere else and what's going to happen next. These might all be valid concerns, but every now and then we need to blank them out, and savour the here and now. You might be able to look at the photos forever, but you'll never have that moment again.

Living your life in more than one gear is a skill you can learn. Sure, there are days when you speed along in the fast lane, but also you need to know when to pull over and enjoy the view. It might be when you're sharing a special time with friends or family, when you've accomplished something that you're proud of or when you just consciously decide to take stock of the good things you've got going on. We spend far too long worrying about what's lacking in our lives without noticing what we already have. Can you really expect more if you don't appreciate what you've got?

The power of three

Try listing three things you're grateful for at the start or end of every day. I'm not a religious person, but I do know to be grateful for what I have, whether that's my health, my job or the people who are in my life. I really believe that positivity creates positivity. When you feel good, good things happen. It's not a mystical thing, it's because you're open to experiences, alert to opportunities and motivated to make changes.

Start a gratitude book

A gratitude book is great way of focusing on the positive. For some years now, I've been jotting down notes on the good things that happen, problems I've overcome, little things that I notice give me pleasure, my strengths and achievements, and things I'm looking forward to. I take note of the good things about the people around me and what I most appreciate about them. A gratitude book helps you train yourself to look at things positively, but flicking through it also gives you a real boost when you do feel blue. Practise gratitude daily, it will help you build a great attitude!

MY BEGINNINGS

I've developed an approach that helps me live my best life, but of course where we come from is part of who we are as well, so I want to share my story with you. Like most stories, mine begins with family, and my family is as tight-knit as can be. There's my mum, my dad and me, and we always have and always will stick together. I owe so much to my family. They've looked after me and stood by me through every crisis, setback or success I've been through.

I was born in Livingstone, a new town on the outskirts of Edinburgh, and have lived in Scotland all my life. I'm proud to call myself Scottish and loved the idea I was representing my country on *Love Island*. However, like millions of other Scots, my genes tell another story. I'm the product of a multi-ethnic family – and that's an understatement!

My maternal grandfather was from Burma (now called Myanmar). At 16 years of age he was working on the container ships taking sugar around the world, and Glasgow was one of his ports of call. The story goes that one day during shore leave he went into a shop, where he met a girl. He fell instantly in love and jumped ship in order to be with her. It's such a fabulously romantic tale – and I'm so proud that my parents gave me his name, Maung, as my middle name.

My grandmother's parents had originally come from Pakistan, so she was also from an immigrant family. They eventually married and went on to have six kids, five of them boys, but the eldest a girl, Sherie Ann, my mum. Like others from Asia, they took advantage of the Scots' growing love of curry and set up an 'Indian' takeaway, the whole family working together in the business.

By 1988, my father was running a pizza delivery service. He too was the child of immigrants: his father had come to Scotland from the Ukraine (hence the name Danyluk) after the end of the World War II, while his mother was Italian. Yep, if anyone has a claim to be multi-ethnic, it's me – each of my grandparents came from a completely different part of the world.

It was time for another love story. In an industrial estate in Livingstone, my dad was working hard on his pizza business. He struck up a friendship with the guy in the next-door unit – an Asian takeaway service – and soon noticed the girl chopping onions in the kitchen. Just like his own father, he fell in love instantly and never looked back.

I OWE SO MUCH TO MY FAMILY. THEY'VE LOOKED AFTER ME AND STOOD BY ME THROUGH EVERY CRISIS, SETBACK OR SUCCESS I'VE BEEN THROUGH.

After they married, mum and dad set up their own popcorn business. They were still working hard to get it up and running when I came along in 1994. I was a happy little boy, often playing with my cousins, but I really can't remember too much about those early days. When I was five, we moved out of Livingstone. It was just 15 or so miles down the M8 towards Glasgow, but it was a different world. My parents had bought an old 30-acre farm in the middle of the countryside, from which they could run the business and where we all could live. It was called Raiziehill Farm, but they named it 'The Ranch'.

This was where I grew up and where I still live. It was and is idyllic. There's plenty of open space and even stables where we used to keep ponies. I was an only child and was – and still am – treated like my parents' most precious treasure ever. They always had time for me, even though they were so busy working, and when they didn't, I'd spend my time with my gran (my mum's mum). My gran died in 2012. My mum was devastated, and it hit me hard too.

The only positive was that I became closer to my grandad. He was funny, quite a Jack the Lad, so maybe I get that side of my character from him. When I was 10 we all went to Myanmar to see where he grew up. It was such an eye-opener to see real poverty, but also that, despite their hardships, people had a dignity and could be happy with so little. And, for a young lad, watching the Water Festival where everyone soaks each other was just fantastic. I was so happy to be able to pay for my grandad to return to the country again once I had earned some money.

WHEN I WAS GETTING INTO TROUBLE AT SCHOOL, MUM WAS THE ONE WHO SAT ME DOWN AND SAID, 'ENOUGH IS ENOUGH – IT'S TIME TO SORT YOURSELF OUT.'

All through my life my mother has remained my best friend. She suffered many miscarriages before having me and lost a brother in a car crash. Whether that meant she took extra care of me I'm not sure, but she always has my back. I tell her everything, including all that goes on with my girlfriends. That can mean she judges them harshly some times. Once a girl I had been seeing for a few months was over at the Ranch and managed to get a quiet word with my mum. She made the mistake of asking what she thought of her and got an honest answer: she was 'five out of ten at best', my mum said, and wasn't good enough for me. That relationship didn't last much longer and it didn't take a lot of hindsight for me to realise mum was right!

I know she will do anything for me. She arranged for me to join a fitness boot camp team which booked a space at the Ranch and she won over the agents who eventually got me on to *Love Island*. We have a real laugh together too and, yes, she still shaves my bum! It's weird how that became such a massive thing when she said it on *Love Island*, as it always seemed pretty normal to us at home. She started doing it when I was earning some cash as a sexy butler. She'd do it every couple of weeks and it really was no bother, but that's just a sign of how close we are.

She refers to herself as a helicopter mum who, when she sees me in need of help, flies down and picks me back up. That's not to say she can't show tough love too when needed. When I was getting into trouble at school, she was the one who sat me down and said, 'Enough is enough – it's time to sort yourself out.' When being overweight was getting me down, she got me up and made me go to the gym every morning before school. And when I came back from *Love Island* and was partying every night, it was Mum who helped me focus on what I really wanted to do, saying, 'You're wasted as a reality star!'

When she appeared on the *Love Island: Aftersun* show, my mum became a bit of a star herself. The nation saw the side of her I'd always known. She was caring, funny, strident and not scared of saying what was on her mind and people instantly warmed to her. She tells it how it is, bigging me up like the loving mum she is, but also calling me out when she felt I was out of order – when I watched it later, I was relieved she wasn't there to scold me for kissing Anna!

My dad is the ying to my mum's yang. He's reserved, laid-back and easy-going, and, unlike Mum, he's not in the least bit scary. That's not to say he won't offer his opinion when he thinks it's necessary and it's always worth listening to when he does. I've learned a lot from him about living your life with dignity. He has set a perfect example in how he treats my mum and other women, and he is always courteous to everyone. I like to think I've learned this from him.

That was how it was at the Ranch – just the three of us. My parents worked intensely hard to grow their business. Even though they barely had the money, they paid for me to go to school, because they felt that was important. Meanwhile, they were giving me the best education possible by bringing me up to be positive, respectful and hard-working and to help others – a set of values that have made me the man I am.

Fitness

Exercise is the keystone to your wellbeing. The benefits of being fit are not limited to keeping your body healthy, but also help you feel better and live a more fulfilled life. Here is what you need to know about being active.

9. Discover fitness

Unlocking the benefits of training transformed my life. It was the key to feeling healthy, self-confident and positive – and looking good. My passion and purpose became to help others find that key.

I love training. It's the thing I look forward to when I get up in the morning and I can't remember a single time when I've regretted going for a workout. I have also been in the business long enough to know that not everyone feels the same. People can become disillusioned, suffer injuries or just get bored and end up dropping out – missing out on a key element of leading their best life. To inspire and help people find that same enduring passion for exercise, no matter what age or stage they are at in their life, became my goal.

My fitness philosophy is born a decade's experience in the fitness industry. I've led classes in many different styles, from body pump to boxing, cardio to boot camp, and after teaching thousands of sessions I came to realise people failed to engage or progress in their fitness goals because they lacked the key elements of concentration, coordination and balance. As a result, I developed my own personal philosophy of how to change not only your body but your mindset as well.

Why keep fit?

I think everyone knows how vital it is to be fit. Regular exercise improves our overall health, including our respiratory (breathing) and cardiovascular (heart) health, and it gives us strong muscles and bones, which can help protect us against osteoporosis (weak, easily fractured bones). This is important not just for now, but for the future, because keeping ourselves fit can also help us maintain a healthy weight and reduce our risk of getting type 2 diabetes, heart disease and some cancers in later life.

The ultimate objective is to complete any exercise you do with perfect form, breathing, posture and timing, and to maximise your workout with minimal effort. By controlling your movements, and learning to contract and squeeze your muscle groups in a way which stimulates more muscle fibre recruitment, you strengthen your muscles and increase the calories you burn.

Having said that, you need to get the basics right. This ensures that, when it comes to stepping up the workouts through weights, reps and/or intensity, you do it safely and effectively. I believe that if we get the basics right and develop the fundamental principles of training, then people will be prepared and inspired to take their fitness to another level.

Training to lose

To help them lose weight, many people look to aerobic exercise, like running, cycling or swimming, that raises the heart rate. This is a good idea, because it burns through the calories pretty rapidly and does wonders for your heart. However, fewer people look to lose body fat through weight training, even though this is a really effective way of doing it, with much less chance of injury. Muscles are an active tissue which, when the body is at rest, burn more energy than fat does. Build your muscle, and you'll build your capacity to burn fat. This is often described as turning your body into a 'fat-burning machine', because it will go on burning that fat when you're back at your desk or lounging around. Think of it in terms of aerobic exercise acting like a microwave that gives short, sharp results, whereas weight training is more like ongoing slow cooking at a low heat.

10. The training basics

I've spent many (happy) years training people outside. You don't need a gym or fancy equipment to perform exercises that will build muscle, make you feel fitter and could even help lose weight.

The easiest way to begin strength training is by using nature's own gym machine: gravity. Bodyweight training, as it's known, is free and on your doorstep (well, even closer), and is the most effective training for beginners and those looking to improve their general fitness. Because you're working the body against the resistance of gravity, the only specialist equipment you need are items commonly found in any home.

A routine of just 20 minutes or so, performed two or three times a week, is enough to build functional strength (joint moves that occur in everyday life) and trigger fat burning. The routine can consist of simple exercises such as press-ups, squats, lunges, crunches and jumping jacks, which are familiar to most people. This is one of the safest types of exercise, because you're in control of your own actions and you can adjust the 'load' with a simple body movement.

Benefits of bodyweight

Most common bodyweight exercises fall under the general title of compound exercises. This means they are movements that work several muscle groups simultaneously. The advantages of these are that they are a time-efficient way of exercising the whole body, improving muscle co-ordination and maximising the calorie-burning effects of exercise.

Importantly, they also provide a great foundation for good training practice. Establishing the right principles for training will help you exercise safely, correctly and effectively.

Principles for training

Always warm-up: Before every session, get the heart pumping with a warm-up of jogging on the spot and some gentle dynamic (continually moving) stretches.

Follow the correct form: 'Form' is the correct method of performing an exercise that ensures it's safe and effective. Keep to simple exercises and, even if you think you know how to do it, follow a reputable YouTube video to make sure you understand the correct form.

Concentrate: Don't rush your exercise. Perform each move slowly and properly. Concentrate on getting the form right before you push yourself.

Regulate your breathing: Take deliberate deep breaths that you can feel flowing through your lungs and exhale smoothly through your mouth.

Focus: Stay in the zone for the entire exercise period. Don't allow your mind to wander. Imagine the muscles contracting and relaxing. It will make you feel stronger and work with more intensity.

Rest: Try to give yourself at least a day between training sessions. This will give your muscles time to recover and strengthen.

Keep progressing: Continually challenge yourself to improve by setting yourself small, achievable goals such as repeating each exercise an extra couple of times or, where possible, making it a little more difficult.

11. Cardio workouts

If you're looking to maintain fitness, lose weight, get ripped or generally stay happy and healthy – which should include just about everyone – you need some regular cardio in your life.

When we say 'cardio' we mean cardiovascular exercise. That's anything that increases your breathing and heart rate – from carrying the shopping home to running the 100 metres. There's a good reason doctors bang on about the need to do regular exercise that raises the heart beat: it strengthens your heart (well, after all, it is a muscle), lowers blood pressure, helps keep bones healthy, makes your lungs stronger and has a host of mental health benefits, including reducing stress and the chances of experiencing depression.

Fat-burning monster

Of course, the main reason many of us love cardio is that it burns the calories. If really you go at it, you can get through 500 calories in just half an hour. That could be a quarter of your daily intake! You don't have to do cardio to lose fat – you could reduce your calorie intake and do resistance training – but when you have a fat-burning monster inside you, why not unleash it?

There are many types of cardio activity but they fall into two categories: LISS (low-intensity steady state) aerobic activities that you can sustain for an extended period of time, such as cycling, swimming or running at a steady pace, and HIIT (high-intensity interval training), which includes sprints, circuit training and similar exercises which leave you breathless within a minute. Which is better for burning fat? Expert views differ, because HITT might burn more calories per minute, but LISS can be performed for an extended period of time, so you'll burn the calories eventually.

Enjoy it!

The truth is… the best form of cardio for you is the kind you enjoy and that works for you. You might like getting out in the open air for a run and find the intensity of a HIIT activity hard to take. Alternatively, perhaps you love the adrenaline burst of a short, sharp sprint but find a drawn-out run a real slog. You've got to enjoy it if you're going to stick with it. It should fit in with your lifestyle, be appropriate for your personal goals and be a pleasure, not a chore.

How much cardio exercise you do depends on what your goals are. You should look at doing a few sessions of 30 minutes or so of moderately intense activity each week, just to keep up healthy fitness levels. However, if you're looking to lose weight and controlling your calorie count in order to do that, you might want to increase the time you spend on the activity or how often you do it, and HIIT sessions are definitely useful if you've got a busy schedule.

For what it's worth, here's my take on cardio. I like to do 30 minutes a day and increase that to 45 minutes to an hour if I'm cutting calories. It feels good to get the body moving, so I like to start the day on the cross-trainer in the gym (I find running puts too much pressure on the joints). I really hate HIIT. When I've done sessions before, I found I was dreading it, but then I discovered boxing training. It's a really great form of cardio. I love it and the high intensity doesn't faze me. That's the perfect type of cardio. For you it might be cycling or swimming, spin or circuits, but the important thing is that you're pushing yourself and burning through those calories without even noticing.

12. Build muscle mass

Developing your muscles is not about vanity. Or, at least, it's not only about vanity! If you want to be stronger, stand tall and feel better about yourself, get on board for some progressive overload.

There are many reasons to build muscle with weight training. You might want to feel stronger, improve your sporting ability, protect your body, increase your metabolic rate to aid weight loss or just make life a little easier. However, building muscle requires more than just visiting the gym and going through the motions – you'll need to push those muscles to their limits.

Your body adapts pretty quickly to the demands you make on it. If your muscles are used to dealing with the exertions of your current training routine, they aren't going to change unless you make them change. Altering your body shape requires continual adjustment to your training and an incremental increase in your workload. By increasing the stress usually placed on your muscles, you're breaking down the fibres, which then rebuild stronger than before. They call it progressive overload, so make your workout that little bit tougher and you will force your body to respond.

Changing up

There are different ways in which you can change up, depending on what you ultimately want to achieve. Increasing the weight or level of resistance will help hypertrophy (building bigger muscles), increasing the number of reps or sets can strengthen muscles and reducing the rest time between sets is a way of increasing muscle endurance.

Taking yourself out of your comfort zone may be necessary, but it doesn't make it easy. Give yourself a fair chance of success by setting targets which you know are achievable. Step up your training with small increments just once a week or even once a fortnight, perhaps adding a couple of reps to each set. Be prepared to postpone a change if it really is too difficult – better to carry on until you're ready to try again than to give in. You also have to be patient, as the most muscle mass you can expect to gain is up to a kilo or so (about two pounds) a month, and for all the sudden gains there will be times when you plateau and don't see very much growth at all.

Eat and sleep

Ensure your diet is sufficient to provide the energy needed for muscle growth, which will probably be a 5% increase on your usual calorie intake. The essential amino acids in protein make it the key muscle-building nutrient, so the extra calories should come from protein-heavy foods such as lean meat, fish and eggs or maybe a protein shake. You should aim to have a protein-based meal a few hours before or within two hours of your training.

Deep sleep is when the magic happens, as your body takes this opportunity to repair muscle fibres and increase muscle mass. Be thankful there's a vital part of the process in which you don't have to do anything except get plenty of shut-eye!

You probably won't lose weight by building muscles, because muscle is much denser than body fat. In fact, you may find that if you lose body fat and gain muscle your weight increases, but that doesn't mean your body won't change shape as, kilo for kilo, muscle takes up less room than fat on your body.

Weight-training terms

Form: Performing the exercise correctly and moving through the full range of motion in your joints using an appropriate weight.

Reps: The performance of one complete exercise that lengthens and contracts a muscle though its range, such as one biceps curl. So 10 reps means repeating the action 10 times.

Sets: The performance of a number of reps without a break. Two sets of 12 squats means you will do 12 reps, rest and then perform another 12.

Rest: The time spent at rest between sets in order for the muscle to recover. This can range from 20 seconds to two or three minutes depending on the severity of the exercise.

13. Resistance training

Simple weight training – or using weights to create resistance – is open to everyone, whether you have access to machines at the gym or some small hand weights at home, and it can open positive transformations in everyone's life.

Put any images of bulging biceped, vein-throbbing, super-strong bodybuilders out of your mind. When I talk about training, I'm thinking of ordinary men and women of all ages and sizes using exercise to strengthen their muscles.

Resistance training just means giving your muscles something to work against to build their strength, endurance and size. The simplest way of doing this is by using your bodyweight to work against your muscles in exercises like press-ups and lunges. If you need to introduce extra weight you could invest in a resistance band or some light dumbbells, although often a couple of tins from the kitchen can be a perfectly good substitute. If you're a beginner at the gym, bypass the free weights and head for the weight machines. These have clear instructions and are much safer to use.

Actually, I know some women steer clear of using weights for fear they will end up looking like the Hulk, but it's a complete myth. If you're female, your body fat, especially breast and hip tissue, and your low level of testosterone, which is the primary muscle-building hormone, both make it virtually impossible for you to develop a muscly physique without going to extremes of diet, supplements and training.

Multiple benefits

There is plenty of scientific research to prove that training even at a low to moderate intensity can make you feel better in a general sense. It helps you to sleep, raises your energy levels, promotes mental sharpness and has a positive effect on your mood by lowering stress and anxiety.

It's amazing how much better you can feel just by carrying a heavy bag with ease, being able to bend down to tie the laces of your trainers or reach up to get that item from the top shelf. Over a period of time, you will also find that resistance training using weights can change your posture and your body shape. Strengthening your core muscles will enable you to sit and stand more upright, and losing body fat will make your muscles appear more defined.

Getting started with weights

1. **Plan your session** to ensure you work all muscle groups.

2. If you're beginning with the machines at a gym, go for the seated leg press, lat pull-down, triceps and biceps cable bars, chest press and shoulder press.

3. **Don't start a rep cold.** Start with 50% of the weigh you plan on lifting and then increase it to 75% before beginning your intended number of reps.

4. A beginner should look to performing 1–2 sets of 8–12 reps on each exercise.

5. **Control the motion.** Inhale and hold your breath as you lift the weight in a strong and forceful manner, exhaling only over the top part of the movement. Then lower the weight under control as you breathe in.

6. **Start with a weight you can comfortably manage** and concentrate on using the correct technique for each exercise. Your last two reps of each set should be a struggle, but you should also be able to maintain form.

7. Reverse the direction smoothly at the bottom position without bouncing the weight as it comes to rest. With practice this will become second nature.

8. **Rest between sets for 60–90 seconds.** As your muscles fatigue during a set, they need time to clear metabolic by-products such as hydrogen ions and lactate.

14. Body definition

Get the arms, shoulders, legs or butt you dream of through training! OK, maybe that's too much to expect, but with a little dedication you can give your body more shape.

So here's the first 'definition' you need to know. 'Toned' might describe a look, but there is no such thing as 'toning' muscles. Muscles can grow or they can shrink, that's it. People use the word 'toned' to describe that hard-muscled, lean-bodied look, but those muscles aren't sculpted, they are built and revealed.

We've all got muscles. We've all got subcutaneous fat too – that's the fat stored just beneath your skin, which you can pinch with your thumb and forefinger. It's this fat which affects what your muscles look like from the outside. Here, then, is the conundrum. Building muscles requires energy, plenty of it. How do you get that energy? Through calories. Giving those hard-earned muscles a defined look, however, means you need to lose the fat that masks them. How do you lose fat? By cutting back on those very calories. But if you lose weight by cutting calories, you'll lose a similar percentage of weight from your muscles as you do from fat (as well as some water weight).

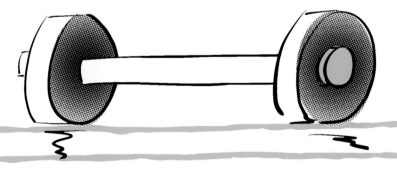

Bulking up

Now, some body builders will take on this challenge. In the off-season, they bulk up by increasing their calorie intake in small increments to build muscle. Inevitably they also put on fat as well, but as competition time comes round they cut calories to lose this fat while working out pretty intensively to maintain their muscle. It's a full-time job, but a short-term fix to the conundrum. I've used this method myself when I've wanted to look my best on the beach on holiday and before I went on *Love Island*.

The bulking route is quite extreme and understandably not for everybody. The more palatable and healthier approach is to lose fat and gain muscle steadily over a longer period. Aim to lose a very small amount – perhaps just a kilo/about 2 pounds – of body fat each month and work on strengthening rather than building your muscles. Remember that you won't lose weight, but depending on your natural shape and your genetic make-up, I promise you'll see changes over time.

Tips for a toned look

▶ Make sure you fit in at least **two weight sessions a week.**

▶ If you're cutting calories, **don't cut the protein.** In fact, try to increase it to at least 30% of your calories.

▶ **Up the cardio sessions** to burn the calories. HIIT workouts may be hard, but they're effective and guard against muscle loss.

▶ **Increase your reps per set** to strengthen muscle and increase the resistance to build muscle.

▶ **Don't concentrate on just one part of your body**. Make sure you hit all the large muscle groups.

Workouts

Working out is central to my life and, ultimately, I couldn't be happy if I wasn't healthy. I believe that everyone feels more fulfilled when they're fit, so I've put together eight progressive workouts that will really set you up for good health.

The following workouts cover cardio, resistance and muscle building, and I've given you clear instructions explaining how to do each individual exercise, as it's vital to get the right form. That's because the right form will not only stop you from hurting yourself, it will also maximise the effectiveness of any exercise.

Of course, to get the right form you can work with a trainer at the gym or at home. They will be able to help you understand exactly how to use your body and get rid of bad habits. However, if you're not ready for that yet, you can also watch videos that will help you hone your technique. There are so many people providing training content online, so find two or three that you like and whom you trust.

In general, for all these exercises, you should inhale when you lift and exhale when you lower. If you're not sure about this, again, watch a video of an expert doing it. Always engage the area of the body that you're working on – try Googling if you're not sure exactly which muscles you're dealing with – and if you do these workouts correctly, you'll enable your core muscles to do their job, which is to protect your spine.

And just a reminder about avoiding injury. It doesn't have to take long, but do warm up. Attempt exercises only when you are clear about how to do them and listen to your body – yes, you want to feel the burn, but not the crash. Always allow your muscles time to recover between sessions and don't overtrain.

What equipment do you need?

I've kept it really simple. A lot of the exercise in these workouts don't require any equipment at all, but a number of them call for dumbbells and there are few that need a kettlebell or band. These can all be bought cheaply for the cost of a month's gym membership. Having said that, though, if you don't have any dumbbells, don't let that stop you. Instead, you can use packets of rice or beans, tins, bottles of water or laundry detergent, or even books.

If you lack a resistance band, you could improvise one from a bungee or, failing that, the tie of a dressing gown. Of course, a proper mat for floorwork is good, but if you're at home you can always use a rug.

They don't have to be fancy, but I would suggest you wear decent gym shoes that provide good support for the arches of your feet and have a cushioned heel to absorb shock. And while it can be nice to have nice clothes, just wear something reasonably loose and comfortable, which gives you room to move and breathe. And that's it. Get the above items sorted and you're all set up.

WORKOUT 1: IN A HEARTBEAT

This is a 25-minute cardio workout, so it's a good one if you're struggling for time. Do the exercises one after another in a circuit format and complete the circuit five times. Perform each exercise for the given number of seconds, then rest for the given number of seconds.

Beginner: 20 seconds' work, 40 seconds' rest

Intermediate: 30 seconds' work, 30 seconds' rest

Advanced: 40 seconds' work, 20 seconds' rest

Exercise 1: High knees

This type of circuit training is high-intensity interval training (HIIT) and you should work as hard as you can before taking the short rest.

1. Stand with your feet hip-width apart.

2. Lift each knee in turn to near chest level and run – or better, sprint – on the spot.

3. Pump your arms to help your balance.

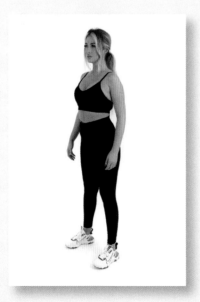 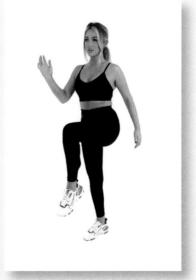

Exercise 2: Squat jumps

The reason you should work as hard as you can is because this increases your Basal Metabolic Rate (BMR), which will help you burn fat for up to 24 hours after the workout.

1. With your feet slightly more than hip-width apart, take up a squatting position. Your butt should be at about knee level.

2. Jump up explosively, using your arms to propel you.

3. As you land, return to the squatting position, again using your arms to help you move.

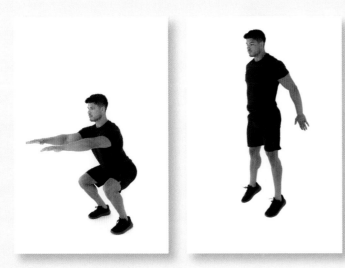

Exercise 3: Press-ups

Don't pace yourself on this circuit. Work full out on each exercise, have a brief rest and then really go for it again, because otherwise you won't get the same metabolic effect. If you can't perform a full press up on your toes, drop to your knees.

1. Lie face down with your legs straight, your palms on the floor at chest level and your arms at a 45-degree angle to your torso.

2. Push up to lift your chest, torso and thighs off the ground, maintaining the tension in your torso.

3. Hold this position and then lower your torso back to the starting position.

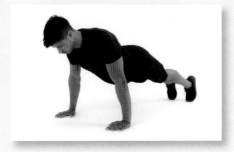
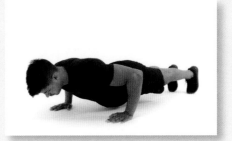

Exercise 4: Plyo lunges

When you get to this exercise for the fourth time you might be flagging, but keep going – and if you're not, then you need to push yourself a bit harder!

1. Stand with your feet shoulder-width apart and step forwards with your right foot.

2. Lower your torso until your right thigh is parallel to the floor and your left knee is almost touching the ground, then explode back up as high as you can.

3. As you land softly, swap legs. Drop straight back into a lunge and then explode back up.

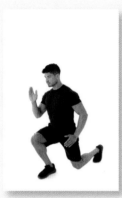 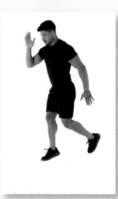 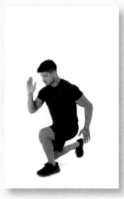

Exercise 5: Burpees

The other good thing about this workout is that it's easy to do at home, because you don't need any special equipment and you don't need a lot of space either.

1. Stand with your feet shoulder-width apart and your arms by your sides.

2. Drop down into a squatting position with your hands on the floor between your knees.

3. Push your legs out behind you, keeping your back straight.

4. Pull your legs forwards, return to a squatting position and then return to the standing position.

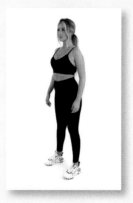 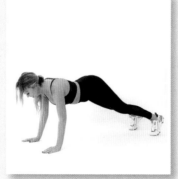 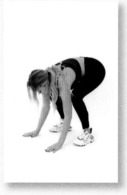

WORKOUT 2: JOIN THE RESISTANCE

If you haven't done resistance or weight training before – and even if you have – this is a great full body workout. Aim to perform it two or three times a week and try to increase the weight at each session, but only if your form is good.

Perform 2–3 sets of 8–12 reps on each exercise

Exercise 1: Goblet squats

In this exercise, make sure you keep the weight close to your body, or it will be much harder to keep your balance and maintain the proper form.

1. Stand with your feet shoulder-width apart. Hold one end of a dumbbell under your chin, palms facing upwards (your hands make the goblet shape).

2. Perform a squat. At the lowest point your elbows should be slightly inside your knees.

3. Return to the standing position.

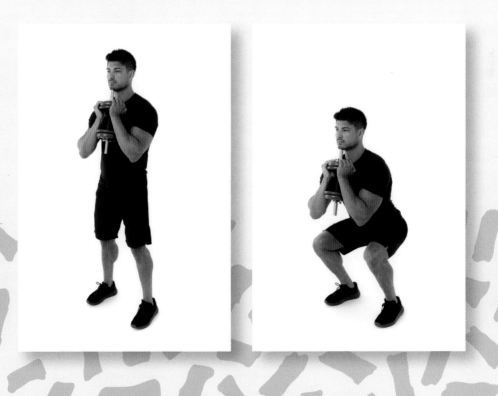

Exercise 2: Dumbbell rows

Your own bodyweight almost always provides some resistance, but in most of the exercises in this workout dumbbells create additional resistance.

1. Stand with your feet hip-width apart, holding a dumbbell in each hand.
2. Bend forwards from the hips, so your back and head are at 45 degrees, and drop your hands down.
3. Squeeze your shoulders together, keep your elbows pointing behind you, and raise and lower the dumbbells.

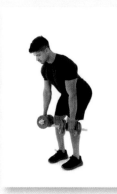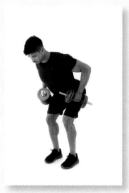

Exercise 3: Dumbbell floor press

Your own bodyweight almost always provides some resistance, but in most of the exercises in this workout dumbbells create additional resistance.

1. Lie on your back with your knees raised until the soles of your feet are flat on the floor.
2. Hold a dumbbell in each hand, just above your shoulders, with your palms facing towards your feet.
3. Extend your arms until they're straight, raising the dumbbells.
4. Lower the dumbbells until your elbows touch the floor.

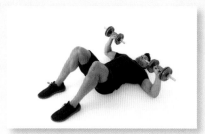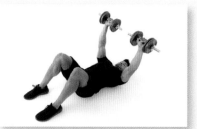

Exercise 4: Standing dumbbell shoulder press

Overhead lifting is a great way to improve your core strength and work the large muscles in your upper body. Remember to pay attention to form and control the dumbbells throughout the set.

1. Stand straight up with your feet around shoulder-width apart.
2. Raise the dumbbells to shoulder height on each side and rotate them so that your palms are facing forwards.
3. Keep your head up and eyes facing forwards. Slowly raise the dumbbells above your head until your arms are almost fully extended.
4. Without pausing, lower the dumbbells back to the starting position.

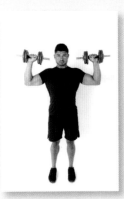 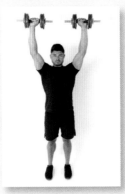

Exercise 5: Dumbbell biceps curls

This is a very simple exercise, which builds strength and definition, particularly in the front of the upper arms, but to a lesser extent in the lower arms as well.

1. Stand with your feet hip-width apart, arms relaxed, palms facing forwards and holding a dumbbell in each hand.
2. Bend at the elbows to raise and lower the dumbbells.

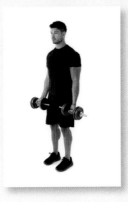 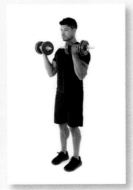

Exercise 6: Dumbbell skull crushers

Perform all these exercises with the correct form (and the right weight, if applicable), and you should really feel the burn on the last few reps.

1. Lie back on the floor, holding a dumbbell in each hand. Raise your arms over your head so the dumbbells are just above your skull. This is the starting position.

2. Straightening your arms, raise the dumbbells.

3. Lift your butt off the floor. Move it forwards slightly, but keep your back close to the floor.

4. Curling your arms, lower the dumbbells.

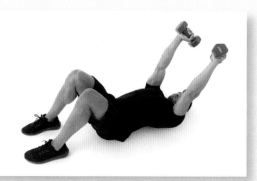 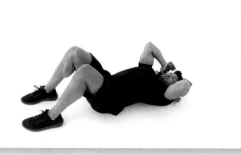

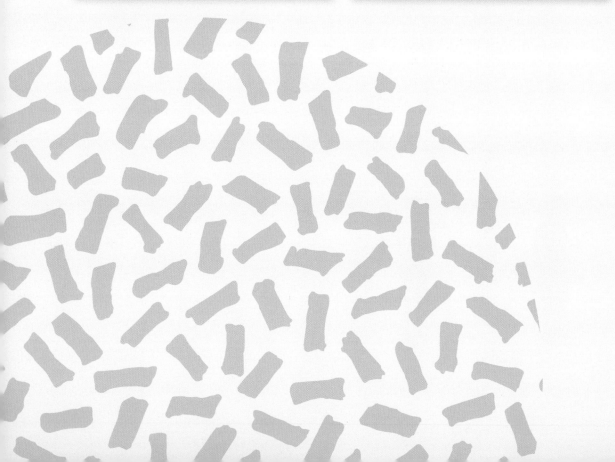

WORKOUT 3: PUT THE KETTLE ON

Here's a full body workout using a kettlebell, but I've broken it down into three separate circuits with each one focusing on a different area – the upper body, lower body and abs. Circuit training is a great way of keeping your heartbeat up and ensuring you maximise the calories you burn in a fixed time, and the kettlebell adds load.

Beginner: 30 seconds on, 30 seconds off, x 2 rounds on each circuit –
60 seconds' rest between circuits

Intermediate: 45 seconds on, 15 seconds off, x 2 rounds x 2 on each circuit –
60 seconds' rest between circuits

Advanced: 60 seconds on, no rest between exercises, x 2 on each circuit –
60 seconds' rest between circuits

UPPER BODY CIRCUIT

Between them these exercises will activate most of the muscles in the upper body, but remember to handle the kettlebell carefully – they're heavy pieces of equipment!

Exercise A: Shoulder presses

1. Stand with your feet hip-width apart. Take the kettlebell in both hands and move it to upper chest level.

2. Push the kettlebell up and over your head. Don't stretch your shoulder out.

3. Return to the starting position.

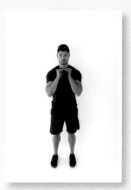 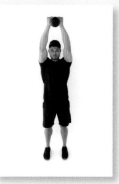

Exercise B: Single arm rows left

1. Stand with your feet shoulder-width apart and place the kettlebell beside your left foot. Take a step back with your right foot and rest your right hand on your right knee.

2. Keeping your spine neutral and your elbow close to your body, raise the kettlebell up to your stomach.

3. Lower the kettlebell.

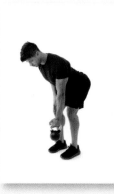 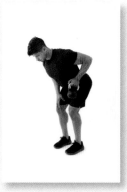

Exercise C: Single arm rows right

1. As above, but switch sides.

Exercise D: Kettlebell press-ups

1. Place the kettlebell on the floor. Lie face down with your legs straight and put one hand on the kettlebell at chest level.

2. Push up to lift your chest, body and thighs off the ground, maintaining the tension in your body.

3. Hold this position and then lower your body back to the starting position.

4. When going through the circuit again change sides.

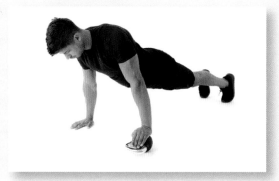 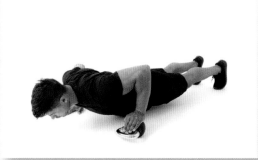

Exercise E: Overhead triceps extensions

1. Stand with your feet shoulder-width apart. Hold the kettlebell in both hands and position it behind your head.

2. Raise the kettlebell above your head, keeping your elbows tucked in.

3. Lower the kettlebell.

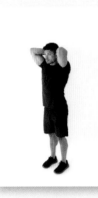 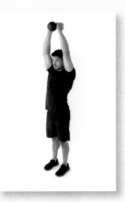

Exercise F: Biceps curls right

1. Stand with your feet hip-width apart, arms by your side, holding the kettlebell in your right hand.

2. Bend your elbows and raise the kettlebell up to shoulder level.

3. Lower the kettlebell by reversing the curl.

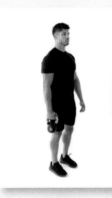 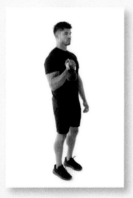

Exercise G: Biceps curls left

1. As above, but switch sides.

LOWER BODY CIRCUIT

The extra load from the kettlebell makes each of these exercises more productive. One safety tip, though – given how heavy a kettlebell is, never do these in bare feet.

Exercise A: Goblet squats

1. Stand with your feet shoulder-width apart. Hold the kettlebell under your chin.

2. Perform a squat. At the lowest point your elbows should be slightly inside your knees.

3. Return to the standing position.

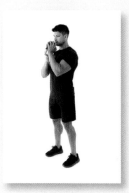 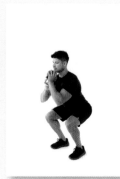 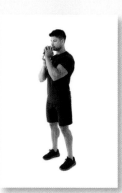

Exercise B: Split squats left

1. Stand with your feet hip-width apart. Take the kettlebell in your left hand so it's by your side.

2. Step back with the left foot. Keeping your hips square and your tailbone tucked under, drop the left knee down and then up again.

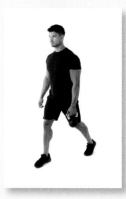 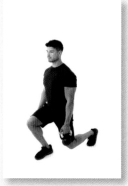

Exercise C: Split squats right

1. As above, but switch sides.

Exercise D: Stiff leg deadlifts

1. Stand with your feet shoulder-width apart, holding the kettlebell in front of you with both hands.

2. Bend your knees slightly and lower the kettlebell over your feet, keeping your back straight and flexing at the hip.

3. Raise the kettlebell.

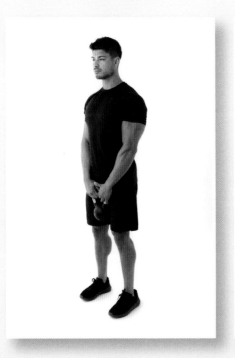
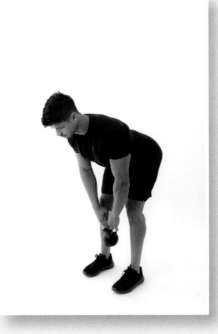

Exercise E: Kettlebell lunges right

1. Stand with your feet hip-width apart, holding the kettlebell at chest height.

2. Lunge forwards with your right leg. Your calf should be at an angle of 90 degrees to your thigh.

3. Push back off the front leg into standing.

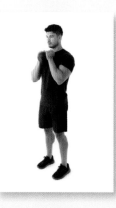
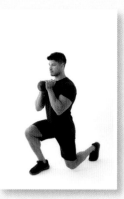

Exercise F: Kettlebell lunges left

1. As above, but switch sides.

Exercise G: Kettlebell hip drives

1. Lie on your back with your knees raised and your feet flat on the floor.

2. Grasp the kettlebell with two hands and fully extend your arms above your chest.

3. Still holding the kettlebell up, raise your hips until they are at an angle of 90 degrees to your lower legs.

4. Lower your hips to the starting position.

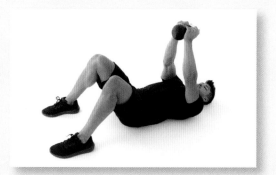
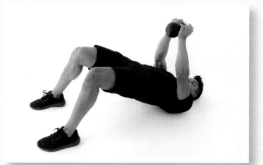

ABS CIRCUIT

Apart from anything else, a kettlebell has a thicker handle than a dumbbell or a barbell, so using a kettlebell will help develop your grip and your forearm strength.

Exercise A: Crunches

1. Lie on your back, knees slightly bent, feet on the floor, holding a kettlebell at chest level with both hands.

2. Keeping your lower back on the floor, tuck your chin in to your chest and use your abdominal muscles to roll your upper back up, so that your body is at an angle of 45 degrees to the floor.

3. Roll back down.

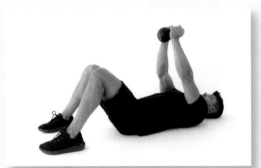 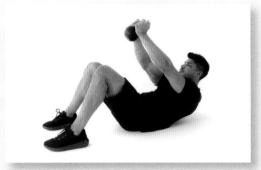

Exercise B: Oblique twists

1. Sit on the floor, knees slightly bent, feet on the floor, holding a kettlebell at chest level with both hands.

2. Rotate your torso as far as you can to the left, return to the centre and then rotate your torso to the right.

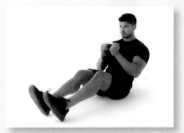 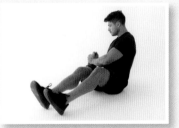 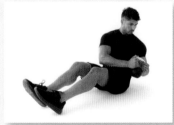

Exercise C: Deadbugs

1. Hold the kettlebell in both hands. Lie on your back with your legs straight and arms extended behind your head.

2. Lift your arms and legs simultaneously until you come into a ball position. Your shoulders should be lifted off the floor.

3. Return to the starting position without letting your legs or shoulders touch the floor.

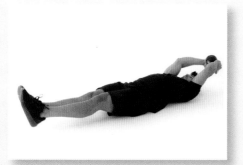 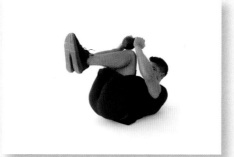

Exercise D: Planks

1. Place the kettlebell on the floor. Kneel in front of it, place your hands on either side of it and straighten your legs out behind you.

2. Raise your body up on to your toes. Keep your spine neutral and look down.

3. Hold this position.

4. Drop to your knees if you can't hold a plank on your toes.

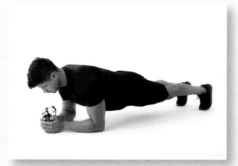 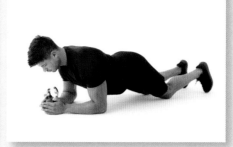

Exercise E: Mountain climbers

1. With your arms extended, both feet pointing forwards and your heels lifted off the floor, bend one leg. Your calf should be at an angle of 90 degrees to your thigh. Extend the other leg backwards.

2. Shift your body weight forwards and switch legs, alternating bending and straightening them.

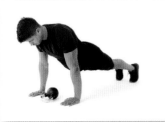 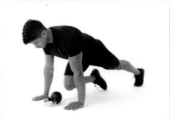 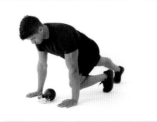

Exercise F: Side planks right

1. Lie on your side with your right elbow below your right shoulder, your legs straight and in line with your body and your feet stacked on top of each other. Take the kettlebell in your left hand, with the bottom of the kettlebell facing upwards, resting the kettlebell on your upper thigh or hip.

2. Raise your body. Keep your spine neutral and your body straight.

3. Hold this position.

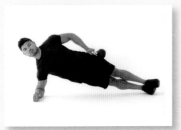

Exercise G: Side planks left

1. As above, but switch sides.

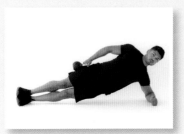

WORKOUT 4: DO THE LEG WORK

If you want to work your muscles harder, switch from full body workouts to sessions that concentrate on either the upper or lower body. The exercises in this lower body workout are grouped into supersets.

Perform 3–4 sets for 8–12 reps on each exercise

SUPERSET 1

The idea of a superset is that you do the two exercises one after another, preferably with no rest in between. This doubles the amount of work you're doing while keeping the recovery period the same.

Exercise A. Goblet squats

1. Stand with your feet shoulder-width apart. Hold one end of a dumbbell under your chin, palms facing upwards (your hands make the goblet shape).

2. Perform a squat. At the lowest point your elbows should be inside your knees.

3. Return to the standing position.

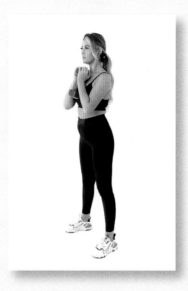 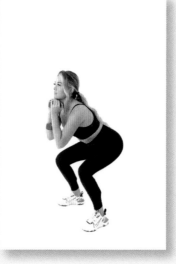

Exercise B. Squat jumps

1. With your feet slightly more than hip-width apart, take up a squatting position. Your tailbone should be just higher than knee level.

2. Jump up explosively, using your arms to propel you.

3. As you land, return to the squatting position, again using your arms to help you move.

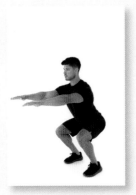 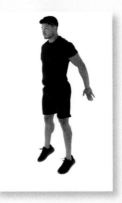

SUPERSET 2

Aim for two upper and two lower body workouts per week, with a rest day between each session. That would look something like upper body sessions on Days 1 and 5, lower body sessions on Days 3 and 7, and breaks on Days 2, 4 and 6.

Exercise A. Dumbbell lunges

1. Stand with your feet hip-width apart, holding a dumbbell in each hand, and step forwards with your right foot.

2. Lower your body until your right thigh is parallel to the floor and your left knee is almost touching the ground.

3. Return to the standing position and repeat by stepping forwards with your left leg.

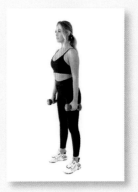 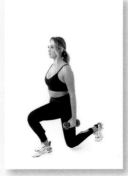 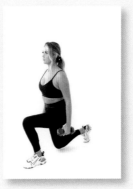

Exercise B. Plyo lunges

1. Stand with your feet shoulder-width apart and step forwards with your right foot.

2. Lower your body until your right thigh is parallel to the floor and your left knee is almost touching the ground, then explode back up as high as you can.

3. As you land softly, swap legs. Drop straight back into a lunge and then explode back up.

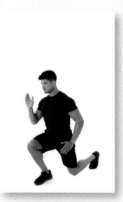 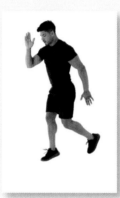 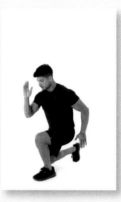

SUPERSET 3

The exercises in this workout all require minimal equipment and if you continue to alternate upper and lower body sessions with rest days, you'll definitely see a difference in four to six weeks.

Exercise A: Stiff leg dumbbell deadlifts

1. Stand with your feet shoulder-width apart, knees slightly bent, holding a dumbbell in each hand.

2. Keeping your back straight, bend at the hips and lower the dumbbells.

3. When you feel your hamstrings starting to tighten, raise the dumbbells up and return to your starting position.

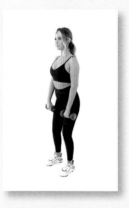 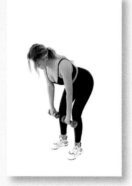

Exercise B: Dumbbell lying leg curls

1. Lie on your front and grip a dumbbell between your feet.

2. Bend your knees back to raise the dumbbell.

3. Lower the dumbbell back to your starting position – without dropping it.

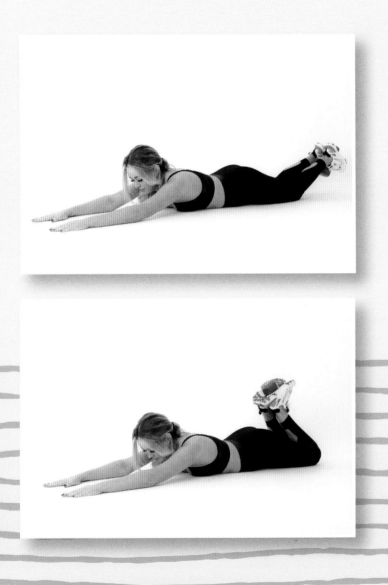

WORKOUT 5: ON THE UPSIDE

You could improvise at home without too much trouble, but for this workout focusing on the upper body it's good if you have a set of dumbbells. Again, it's based on supersets of two exercises, which should be performed back to back, with a minimal – or ideally no – pause between them.

Perform 3 sets for 8–12 reps on each exercise

SUPERSET 1

Go straight from A to B without stopping, but you can take a short 60-second rest to catch your breath after you've completed each of these supersets.

Exercise A: Dumbbell floor press

1. Lie back with your feet firmly on the floor, holding a dumbbell in each hand just beside the lower part of your chest.
2. Start with the dumbbells raised, arms straight.
3. Bend your elbows outwards as you lower the dumbbells.
4. Straightening your arms, push the dumbbells back to the starting position.

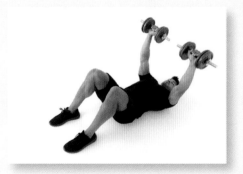 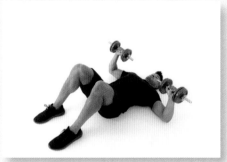

Exercise B: Single arm dumbbell rows

1. Take a step back into a lunge position with your front knee in line with your ankle and your back leg straight. Lean slightly forwards, with the dumbbell-holding arm fully extended downwards and your free hand resting on your front thigh.

2. Push your elbow up and raise the dumbbell to hip level.

3. When you finish the set, repeat with your stance reversed and the dumbbell in your other hand.

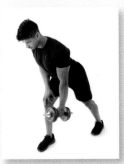 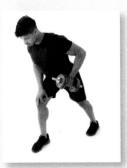

SUPERSET 2

Because the volume of work is higher, your muscles will need time to recover, so do this workout no more than a couple of times per week.

Exercise A: Band chest flies

1. Anchor your resistance band firmly at chest height. Gripping the band handles, stretch it across the back of your shoulders.

2. Move one foot forwards, so you can feel the tension in the band, keeping your leg straight but relaxed.

3. Slowly extend your arms out to the side of your body at shoulder height.

4. Hold briefly before bringing your arms together in front of your chest.

5. Hold briefly before releasing your arms and returning them to the side of your body.

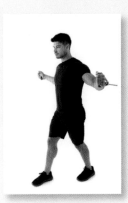 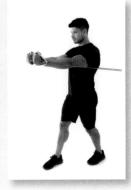

Exercise B: Band high rows

1. Fix the band at chest-height and, facing the band anchor, grasp the handle at arm's length with both hands.

2. With a straight back, pull your elbows back until your hands are in front of your chest.

3. Hold briefly before slowly straightening the arms and returning to the starting position.

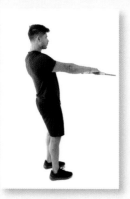 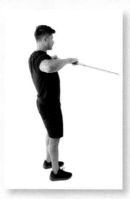

SUPERSET 3

It might be tempting, but don't rest between the exercises in a superset. The aim is to minimise time, but maximise effort and thus results.

Exercise A: Band shoulder presses

1. Stand feet apart on the centre of the resistance band.

2. Hold each handle just above shoulder height, with palms facing forwards.

3. Extend your arms a shoulder-width apart until they are above your head before slowly lowering the band down again.

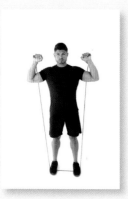 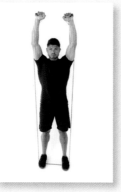

Exercise B: Band lateral raises

1. Stand with one foot on the band (if the resistance isn't strong enough you can use both feet).
2. Start with your arms by your side.
3. Lift your arms to shoulder height, but keep your elbows slightly bent.
4. Return to the starting position.

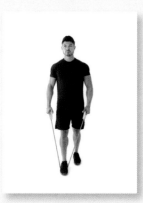
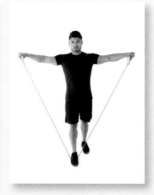

SUPERSET 4

Once you've mastered the workouts that focus on your lower and upper body, you'll be able to zoom in on and work muscle groups in more specific areas.

Exercise A: Band single arm overhead tricep extensions

1. Stand with your feet hip-width apart on one end of the band. Grip the handle of the band and raise it to behind your head.
2. Keeping your head and back straight, extend your arm above your head until it's almost completely straight. Then return your hand to the starting position behind your head.
3. Repeat the set with the other hand.

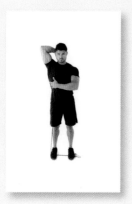
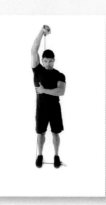
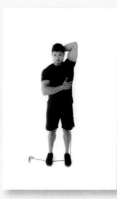
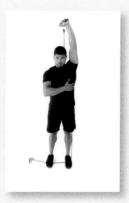

Exercise B: High biceps band curls

Resistance bands are ideal for bicep exercises because resistance level increases as the band is stretched. This means your muscles face the highest resistance when they are in their strongest position.

Perform 4 sets of 8–12 reps

1. Anchor your band at shoulder to chest height.
2. Position yourself a metre or so back, standing facing the anchor with feet apart.
3. Hold the handles at arms length with the palms facing upwards.
4. Curl your forearms in until your hands almost touch your ears. Return to the starting position.

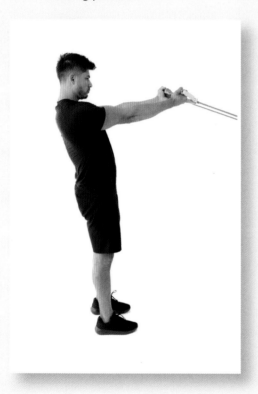 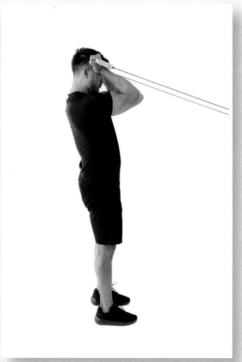

WORKOUT 6: STRONG ARM TACTICS

I recommend you do this workout at least once and preferably twice a week. It's carefully designed to focus on strengthening your arms, so as you go through each of the elements, really concentrate on squeezing and contracting those arm muscles.

Exercise 1: Standing dumbbell biceps curls

Bicep curls are great for speedy improvement in strength and definition. They work not only the biceps muscles at the front of the upper arm, but also the muscles of the lower arm.

Perform 4 sets of 6–8 reps

1. Stand with your feet shoulder-width apart holding a dumbbell in each hand.
2. Allow your arms to hang by your side with your elbows close to your sides and your palms facing forwards.
3. Curl the dumbbells up until they are level with your shoulders.

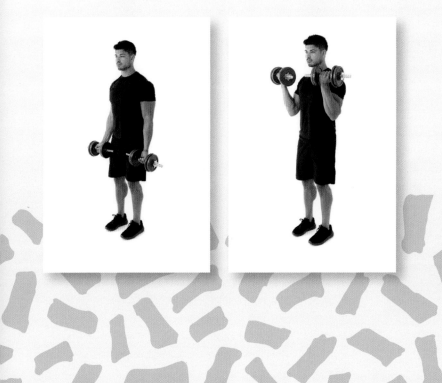

Exercise 2: Standing hammer curls

One of the keys to maximising the effectiveness of this exercise is stationary elbows. Imagine they're glued to your sides or held in place by a vice.

Perform 4 sets of 8–12 reps

1. Stand straight, holding a dumbbell by your side in each hand with palms facing the body.

2. Bend your elbows and raise the dumbbells to shoulder level. Keep your elbows close to your body and don't move them.

3. Lower the dumbbells back to starting position.

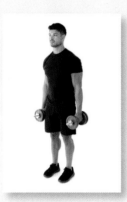 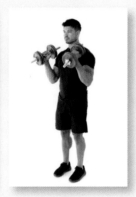

Exercise 3: High biceps band curls

Perform 4 sets of 8–12 reps

1. Anchor your band at shoulder to chest height.

2. Position yourself a metre or so back, standing facing the anchor with feet apart.

3. Hold the handles at arms length with the palms facing upwards.

4. Curl your forearms in until your hands almost touch your ears. Return to starting position.

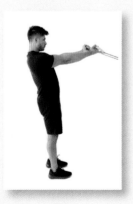 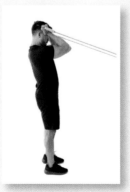

Exercise 4: Close Grip dumbbell floor press

Here 'close grip' means you hold the dumbbells lengthways, parallel to your body, and you push them against each other as you raise and lower them.

Perform 4 sets of 6–8 reps

1. Lie back on the floor, holding a dumbbell in each hand with your elbows resting on the floor. Tuck in tight in line with your lower chest.

2. Push the dumbbells up until they become straight, keep your elbows tight at all times.

3. Lower to the starting position.

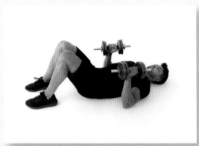 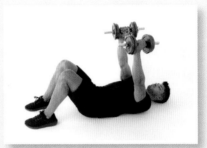

Exercise 5: Dumbbell skull crushers

This exercise zeroes in on strengthening your triceps and it's important because you need strong triceps muscles to complete a range of upper body exercises successfully.

Perform 4 sets of 8–12 reps

1. Lie back on the floor, with your legs slightly bent, holding a dumbbell in each hand. Raise your arms over your head so the dumbbells are just above your skull. This is the starting position.

2. Straightening your arms, raise the dumbbells.

3. Curling your arms, lower the dumbbells.

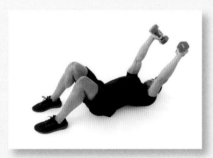 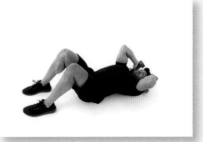

SUPERSET

Remember, a superset ups the intensity, because you go straight from one exercise to the next, with no rest or recovery time in between.

Exercise A: Overhead band extension

1. Lie the band on the floor. Step on it with your feet. Pull the band up behind you with your right hand. Your elbow should be above your shoulder and your hand behind your head.

2. Straighten your arm from your elbow to raise your hand.

3. Lower your hand.

4. Complete the reps, then switch sides.

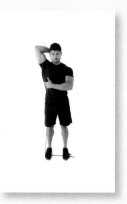 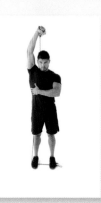 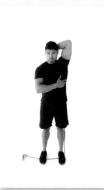 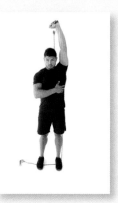

Exercise B: Dumbbell kickbacks

1. Stand leaning forwards with one leg forwards, one leg back and your knees slightly bent, holding a dumbbell on the same side as the leg that is back.

2. From the elbow, bend your arm behind you, keeping it touching your side.

3. Raise the dumbbell back, extending your arm.

4. Lower the dumbbell to the starting position.

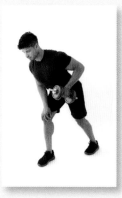 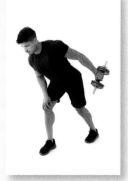 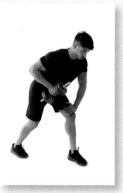

WORKOUT 7: ROCK BOTTOM

As well as focusing on working your butt, this workout is a circuit, so it will also elevate your heart rate and burn a lot of calories too. Do the exercises straight through, one after another, and complete the circuit five times, but you can rest for 60 seconds at the end of each circuit.

Beginner: 20 seconds' work, 40 seconds' rest

Intermediate: 30 seconds' work, 30 seconds' rest

Advanced: 40 seconds' work, 20 seconds' rest

Exercise 1: Glute kickbacks right

I promise you – if you do this workout two or three times a week, it won't be long before you start to see the benefits.

1. Position yourself on all fours, with your back straight.
2. Raise your right leg behind you and up until your thigh is parallel with the floor.
3. Squeeze your glute and hold.
4. Lower your leg back down, but don't let your knee touch the floor.

Exercise 2: Glute kickbacks left

- As above, but switch sides.

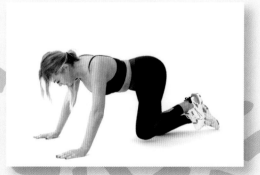 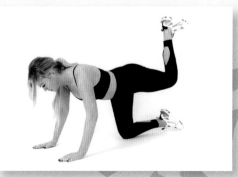

Exercise 3: Hip drives

As with all circuit format workouts, go for it from the start. You need to get your heart beating, which means there's no point in holding back so that you can manage all five rounds with ease.

1. Lie on your back with your feet hip-width apart, your butt resting on the ground and your hands behind your head.

2. Raise your torso up and push your hips forwards slightly, squeezing your butt as hard as you can.

3. Lower your torso back to the starting position.

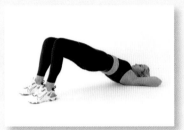 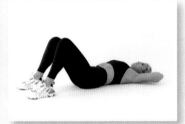

Exercise 4: Squat jumps

If you find this, or any of the other workouts, tough, that's totally to be expected, but don't let it affect your resolve. Each time you do it, you'll get further in before you start to tire.

1. With your feet slightly more than hip-width apart, take up a squatting position. Your tailbone should be just higher than knee level.

2. Jump up explosively, using your arms to propel you.

3. As you land, return to the squatting position, again using your arms to help you move.

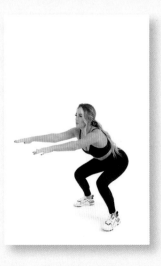 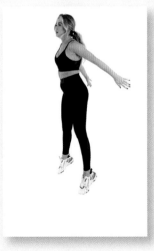

Exercise 5: Plyo lunges

This workout is great for your butt, but it's not just about looking good. Your glutes are a major muscle group and they're essential for explosive movements like sprinting and jumping.

- Stand with your feet shoulder-width apart and step forwards with your right foot.

- Lower your body until your right thigh is parallel to the floor and your left knee is almost touching the ground, then explode back up as high as you can.

- As you land softly, swap legs. Drop straight back into a lunge and then explode back up.

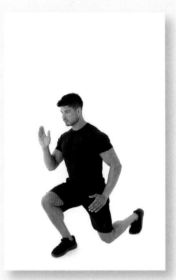
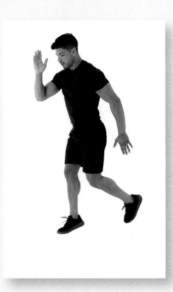
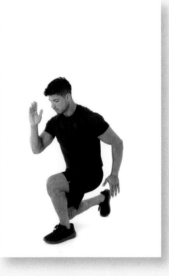

WORKOUT 8: ABS FABULOUS

Here are some more supersets. These target your upper and lower abs, and your obliques. Execute them properly, and they'll do wonders for you. Don't take a break between each group of two exercises, but you can have a 60-second rest between the supersets.

Supersets 1 and 2: perform 3 sets for 10–15 reps on each exercise

Superset 3: perform 3 sets of 45 seconds on each exercise

SUPERSET 1

This whole workout is short, but effective. Do it two or three times a week, and you'll see quick results.

Exercise A: Crunches

1. Lie on your back, knees slightly bent, feet on the floor and hand on your head.

2. Keeping your lower back on the floor, tuck your chin in to your chest and use your abdominal muscles to roll your upper back up, so that your body is at an angle of 45 degrees to the floor.

3. Roll back down.

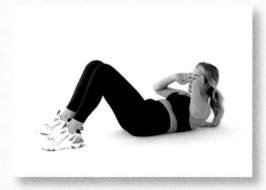 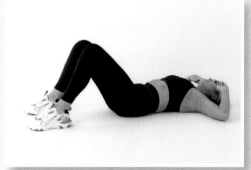

Exercise B: Reverse crunches

1. Lie on your back. Raise your legs so your thighs are at an angle of 90 degrees to the floor and your calves are at an angle of 90 degrees to your thighs (parallel with the floor).

2. Raise your knees up towards your chest and lift your hips off the floor.

3. Lower your legs to the starting position.

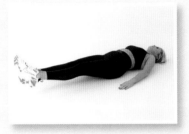 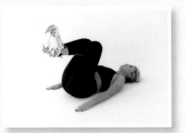

SUPERSET 2

Not only is this workout pretty quick, it doesn't require any special equipment either, so you can do it anywhere.

Exercise A: Russian twists

1. Sit with your legs at an angle of 45 degrees and lean back at an angle of 45 degrees. Hold your arms out in front of your chest and link your hands together.

2. Move your arms to the right, twisting your torso and not moving your head.

3. Move your arms to the left, again twisting your torso.

4. Return your arms to the starting position.

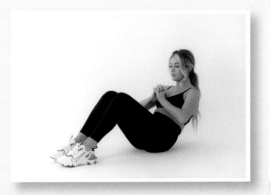 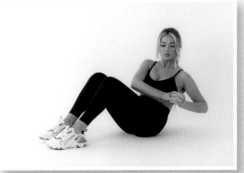

Exercise B: Flutter kicks

1. Lie on your back with your shoulders relaxed and your arms by your side.

2. Point your toes and lift both feet slightly off the ground.

3. Keep your legs straight and begin to raise alternate legs; one leg gently kicking high while the other is lowered.

4. The lowered leg should be no more than 8 centimetres (3 inches) off the floor.

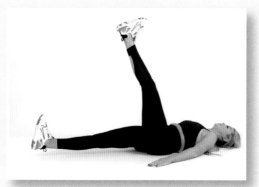 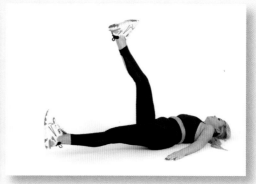

SUPERSET 3

The following two exercises are certainly well-known, but take the time to make sure you know how to do them correctly – as always, the right form is crucial.

Exercise A: Planks

1. Place your hands on the floor, a shoulder-width-apart and move your knees to below your hips.

2. Raise your body up onto your toes. Keep your spine neutral and look down.

3. Hold this position.

4. Drop to your knees if you can't hold a plank on your toes.

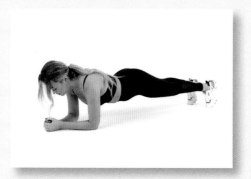 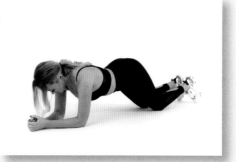

Exercise B: Mountain climbers

1. Place your hands on the floor, shoulder-width apart. With both feet pointing forwards and your heels lifted, bend one leg. Your calf should be at an angle of 90 degrees to your thigh.

2. Shift your body weight forwards and switch legs, alternating bending and straightening them.

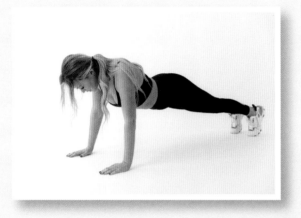

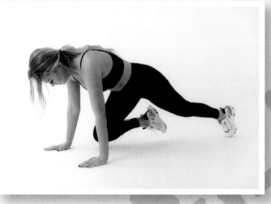

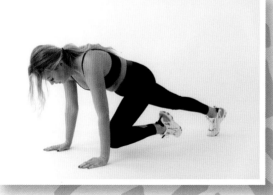

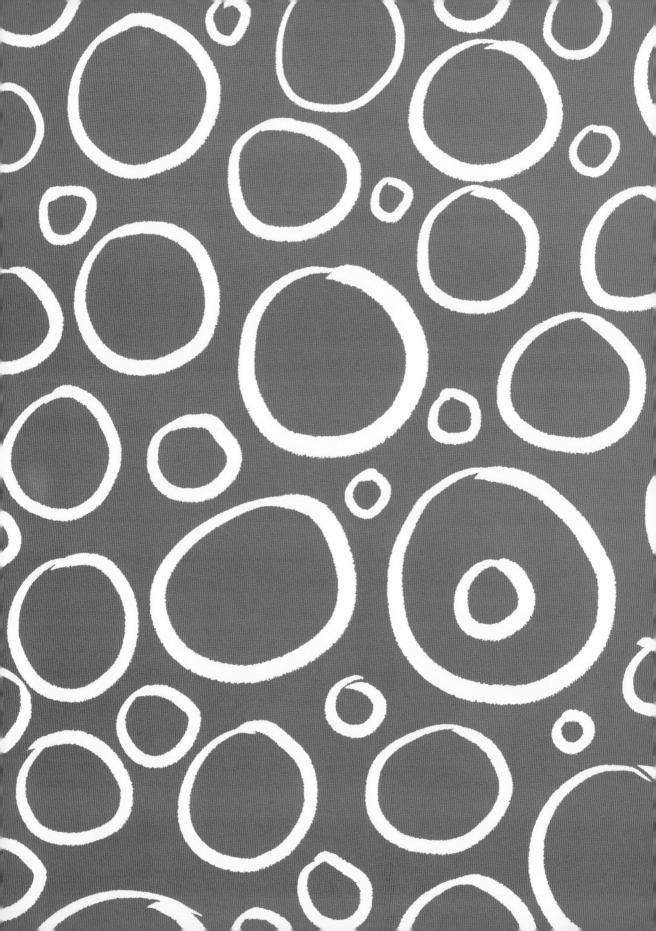

Eating well

Food plays a major part in determining your energy levels, your mood and your overall health, but it isn't difficult to balance each of these requirements – and still lose weight if that's your objective.

15. Losing weight

Losing weight is such a big goal for so many people. It can be difficult, but it doesn't have to be complicated. That's because there are really only two kinds of diet: a surplus calorie diet or a deficit calorie diet.

Type the word *diet* into Google and you'll get 1.2 billion results. There's a lot of interest in losing weight and there's a lot of advice available. I know some people are looking for a super-quick way to drop the kilos, others for a new approach to dieting that might work for them. There are so many options, suggestions and theories out there. It's really not surprising that so many people get confused. For me, though, it's very simple.

Your body needs nutrients for health and calories for energy. The number of calories you need will depend largely on your weight, age and how active you are. If you consume more calories than you need, your body will store it as fat and you will put on weight. If you consume less, it will turn to your fat reserves for energy. To lose weight, the calories you burn through sleeping, everyday life and exercise must be more than the amount you consume. Everything else is window dressing. It may not seem like a magic formula, it isn't a quick fix and it certainly isn't easy, but it works – every time.

Of course, the aim for any weight loss programme is to achieve your ideal healthy weight. That ideal is going to be different for different people, but eating healthily and regularly is important for everyone, and you should always put your long-term wellbeing first.

The basic in/out principle

Each generation has their own favourite weight-loss diets. Ask your parents about the F-Plan, the Grapefruit Diet or Slim Fast meal substitutes. Most of these can help you lose weight, because, however you dress it up, sticking to them will mean your body uses more calories than it consumes. Our generation has taken to intermittent fasting diets such as the 5:2 or the 16/8, when you severely restrict the intake of calories for certain periods. They can be very effective and I have used them myself, but they still work on the same basic in/out principle, so if you pig out too much on your relaxed days, you'll gain rather than lose weight.

Keeping it simple seems like a no-brainer to me. You don't need to buy special products, starve yourself at certain times or exclude certain foods from your diet. All you need is some basic knowledge of (or easy online access to) the number of calories and the nutrients in the food and drink you are consuming, a set of kitchen scales to check your portion sizes and a positive attitude...

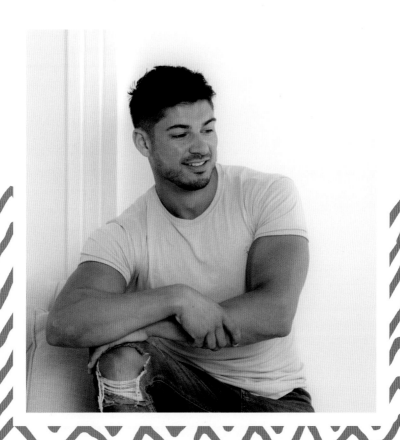

16. Numbers game

You can lose weight. I guarantee it – and I'm not selling some fad diet, I'm going purely on the science and positivity. All you need to do is pay attention to the numbers. Whether you're concerned with maintaining, losing or gaining weight, the details count.

We might all differ in terms of how much we can consume without putting weight on, but our bodies all work in the same way: calories in, calories out. Everyone has their own golden number at which we go into calorie deficit or surplus. Work that out, and you've taken the first step to controlling your weight.

Some simple maths

First, work out your Basal Metabolic Rate (BMR). This is the amount of energy (calories) which your body burns at rest each day. You can find your BMR by using one of the many online BMR calculators or get a reasonable estimation by converting your body weight to pounds and multiplying that figure by 10.

For example, if you weigh 11 stone (70 kg) that's equivalent to around 155 pounds and 155 x 10 = 1550, so your BMR is 1550. This is the number of calories you require to get through a relaxed 24-hour day with 8 hours' sleep and very little activity. However, even couch potatoes get up off the sofa, even if it's just to walk to the corner shop and back. You therefore need to calculate your Total Daily Energy Expenditure (TDEE) – an estimate of how many calories you burn each day, including any exercise you typically take. To do this, take your BMR and multiply that by the amount of exercise you do.

- If you rarely exercise, multiply your BMR by 1.2

- If you exercise on 1 to 3 days per week, multiply your BMR by 1.375

- If you exercise on 3 to 5 days per week, multiply your BMR by 1.55

- If you exercise on 6 to 7 days per week, multiply your BMR by 1.725

- If you exercise every day and have a physical job or if you often exercise twice a day, multiply your BMR by 1.9

You now have your TDEE. If you stick to this, you should not lose or gain weight. These numbers are, of course, estimates. If you find you're keeping to your TDEE, but are losing or putting on weight, then simply add or subtract 100 calories from your daily total until you reach a steady weight. If you're on a weight loss programme, your TDEE will change as you lose weight, add muscle or change your lifestyle. Recalculating your numbers is all part of the fun and can be a great motivator to drive you to your goal.

Use your muscle

Your Basal Metabolic Rate (BMR) is largely determined by your body weight, but other factors come into play too. Although most of these are genetic and out of our control, muscle mass is one variable that does increase the metabolic rate (the speed at which we burn calories). Just as a Range Rover devours more petrol than a Corsa, so a muscular body gets through more calories. Estimates suggest that every pound of muscle burns around six calories per day even at rest, so when you are at the gym, don't focus solely on the cardio machines, but play the long game and use the weights too.

17. Freedom and flexibility

Being able to choose what and when you eat can help you find a diet you can follow and sustain. There are no 'good' or 'bad' foods, just some sensible and healthy choices.

Your diet is just a description of what you eat and drink. It doesn't have to lead to weight loss or gain, doesn't have to entail excluding certain foods and isn't for a limited time only. In order to lose or gain weight you do not need to 'go' on a diet, you need to 'change' your diet. It requires a shift in your lifestyle that will help you reach your optimum weight and stay there.

Chocolate and chips

I follow a flexible diet. I eat and drink when I want and what I want. Absolutely nothing is off limits, including chocolate, chips, fried chicken... Sounds too good to be true? Well, yes and no. I'm aware of the number of calories and amounts of proteins, fat and other nutrients required to get me to, or keep me at, my target weight. As long as I'm hitting those numbers, I have what I feel like. It may mean that if I have a bar of chocolate in the afternoon, I have salad instead of pasta in the evening, or if I have chips one night, I limit myself to soup the following lunchtime, but within my overall calorie count I give myself a lot of freedom.

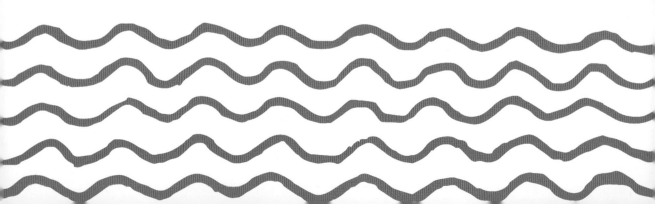

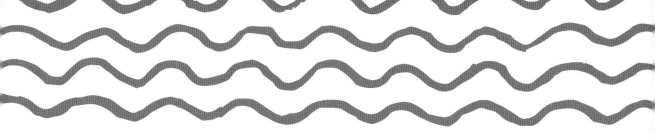

Losing weight isn't easy. If it was, everyone would look trim. With some focus, though, it's definitely possible. You won't see overnight results, but it will be noticeable quite quickly – soon enough to keep you motivated. You should aim to lose only around 1–2% of your body weight per week (except in the first week where water contributes to a large part of the loss). Any more can lead you to lose muscle too, could affect your health and will severely test your will power. For most people this will mean two or three pounds, or just over a kilo, a week – or a stone, or roughly 6 or 7 kilos, in around six weeks.

What my calculations look like

- It takes 3500kcals to burn one pound or half a kilo of fat. Therefore, to burn a pound of fat per week requires a 500kcal deficit on my TDEE per day.

- I weigh 200lb (around 90 kilos), so my BMR is 200 x 10 = 2000Kcals.

- I exercise 6 to 7 days per week, so I multiply the 2000kcals by 1.725, giving me a TDEE of 3450.

- I aim to lose 1% of my body weight a week: 1% of 200 is 2lb.

- To lose 2lbs, I need a deficit of 7000kcals a week or 1000kcals a day.

- My new daily calorie target is now my TDEE (3450) minus 1000.

- I should be able to lose my two pounds a week if I limit my consumption to 2450 calories a day.

So that might sound like a pretty generous daily calorie intake, but remember I'm male, a good weight for me is about 14 stone, and I do a lot of exercise, and those are all factors that affect my numbers and how much I can eat each day if I want to maintain or reduce my weight. If you're female, your numbers are probably going to be quite different, but the basic principles and the approach will be the same.

This applies to women just as much as men, too, and it's important: allow yourself as many calories as you can while still losing weight, so begin with as small a reduction as you can on your TDEE. If you find the weight isn't shifting after a week, drop another 100 calories a day over the following week. If you lose more than 2% of your body weight, increase your calorie allowance by a similar amount. There is simply no point in pushing yourself harder. Without the necessary calories, your body will set itself to survival mode and adjust accordingly. You'll feel listless and won't lose much weight, and if you aren't careful you can enter a negative cycle where you are continually reducing your calorie allowance, and that's not healthy.

Some people, especially those wanting to build their muscles, will need to adjust their diet to gain weight. Bulking, as the bodybuilders call it, follows a similar process as losing weight, but adds rather than subtracts from the TDEE. However, as the aim is to gain muscle and not fat, you should be looking to increase your bodyweight by only 0.5% a week – around 100–200 calories – and you should focus on protein and carbohydrates rather than sugary or fatty foods.

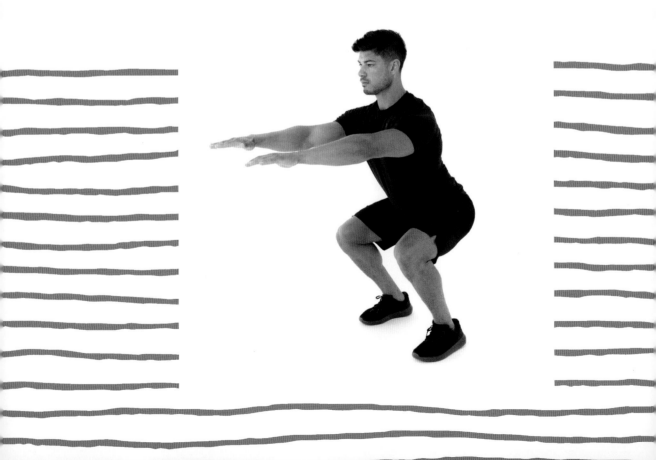

Get on the scales

Not everyone likes the idea of getting on the scales, but it's the best way of monitoring your progress and motivating yourself.

▶ Weigh yourself regularly, but not obsessively. Once a week is enough.

▶ Weigh yourself at the same time (preferably in the morning) and in the same way (with similar clothes or naked).

▶ Invest in a smart scale, which connects to an app on your phone. This will monitor your weight loss as well as keeping a record of your body fat percentage and muscle mass.

▶ Remember, the scales don't lie, but they don't quite tell you the whole truth either. Water and other bodily waste can add pounds, the menstrual cycle can cause weight gain and lean muscle tissue weighs more than fat.

18. Keeping going

Even the most dedicated dieter is going to trip up sooner or later. We're only human. However, with some determination, honesty and a flexible approach, sticking to the plan really isn't that difficult.

This is going to sound brutal but… when you begin your new diet, ask yourself if you can do this forever. If your answer is no, don't start. If you have a target weight, fine, you can ease up when you reach it. Even then, you still need to understand that without changing your lifestyle choices your weight is going to go right back on.

At the same time, though, you need to admit to yourself that it isn't always going to be easy. There will be hard days, times when you give in to temptation and social occasions that put you in a seemingly impossible situation. And there will be weeks when the scales don't budge and you'll wonder whether they ever will. Those are the times to remember why you started the diet, what you wanted to achieve and to have faith in the science – it does work.

Savour your success

There are time-honoured motivations to help you through. Take a photo of yourself when you begin and, wearing the same clothes, take them at regular intervals as you lose weight. Celebrate the milestones – 2 kilos, 5 kilos, 10 kilos – not with food but with clothes, a facial or a trip to the nail bar – and take compliments from friends seriously. In fact, note them down to remind yourself when things get tough.

Of course, slip-ups are going to happen. Maybe in a weak moment you can't resist an unplanned snack or you miscalculate what you've got in the fridge. It's not a disaster. Your calorie allowance doesn't reset at midnight. Use the next day or even the next few days to get yourself back on track. It's really no biggie. Allow yourself to fail once in a while. There's always next week. The worst reaction is to give up and ruin the effort you've already made. Also, the great thing about flexible dieting is that you can even factor in these eventualities. For example, you could decide to 'save' 200 or 300 calories over the week and perhaps have that glass of wine or chocolate bar at the weekend.

Bingeing, cheating and re-feeding

Then there are the days it really goes all Pete Tong. You've built up a 7000-calorie deficit and are on track to dropping a couple of pounds or a kilo. Saturday comes and you just lose it. A medium pizza will deliver over 2000 calories, diving into a tub of ice cream could be at least 300 more and even a single can of Coke or a beer will take you near the 3000 mark. That's how easy it is to consume calories. Now, I'm not saying don't eat junk food or that you should never let yourself have an occasional binge. It all comes down to what you want more and how much you're willing to sacrifice. For you, having that meal might be more important to you than losing weight that week. That's absolutely fine, but you need to work that out for yourself.

A cheat day is a day when you allow yourself to break the rules of your diet in terms of calories, fat or sugar. If you are on a long-term diet, a one-off cheat day might give you something to look forward to and an impetus to continue. Personally, I prefer a re-feed day, which is when you deliberately increase your calorie consumption by increasing your carb intake. This does come as a treat if you're struggling with your allowance, but more importantly it activates the hormones that drive the body's fat burning process. Those hormones can become accustomed to a lower calorie diet and adjust their response accordingly, but they can be also be tricked into thinking your consumption has increased. You should have a re-feed day only once every two weeks and you should increase your calories by around 20%, but for that day only.

Use an app

I'd recommend a weight loss app to anyone seriously monitoring their calories and consumption. They can provide a real boost to your motivation as well as keeping tabs on your calorie intake and tracking weight loss. Apps such as Lose It!, MyFitnessPal, Noom, Fitbit and others make it easy to log what you eat through the day with massive databases of foodstuffs and a simple updating process. They can sync with fitness apps to adjust your calorie requirement according to your daily exercise and can generate reports, graphs and charts that show you your progress. If you haven't used one before, give it a go – an app might just make the difference for you.

19. Food choices

What, when and how much you eat is crucial to maintaining any healthy weight-loss diet. Most of us know by now what's good for us and what's not, but a few tips never go amiss.

I don't want to patronise you by telling you what to eat. Everyone knows the perils of sugar, unsaturated fats and overeating, but here are a few things I've picked up that might help you stick to your calorie allocation.

Help yourself

I get hungry in the evening. I know that by now (in fact, I don't keep food in the house at night – it gets taken to my parent's place), so I plan my eating around a larger carb-based meal later in the day. This means I have to have a low-carb breakfast and a low-calorie lunch, but I find the sacrifice worth it. You might be different. Perhaps you wake up hungry, you like a late snack, you don't mind going to bed early after a light meal or you prefer to spread your calorie intake over the day. That's all fine, as long as you plan ahead and work your consumption around that when you're going to feel hungry.

Cooking my own meals is something I've done from an early age, so I never find it a problem. When you're calorie counting it is extra important, because it means you can control exactly what you're eating. Steer clear of the supermarket low calorie, ready meals because these often have far too much added salt or sugar – and the portions are seldom big enough to stop you wanting something extra later on!

If you don't have kitchen scales, buy some; if you do, use them. For some foods, such as lettuce, broccoli and other leafy vegetables, portion control is not an issue. However, for many carb-, fat-, sugar- or protein-heavy foods, even 10 or 20 grams (1/2 to 3/4 ounces) can make all the difference to your weight-loss plan. More dangerously, not weighing can be a slippery slope, as it's so easy to add a little more to the pan or plate each time without realising it.

The calories in a healthy diet should be made up of 40% carbs, 40% protein and 20% fat, but when you're cutting back, protein is a godsend. It reduces your appetite, boosts your metabolism and is low in calories compared to carb-heavy foods. That means make good use of eggs (any way you like them), fish and chicken, turkey or tofu to fill your plate. This is especially true if you're using resistance training as a part of your programme or are trying to build muscle.

Easy wins

It's worth having a few foods in the cupboard or fridge which you know you can always turn to for a low-calorie easy win. You'll soon be able to work out your own list according to what you find tasty, but mine includes porridge, cod or salmon, boiled potatoes, low-sugar baked beans, turkey strips, veggie burgers and a low-fat avocado oil spray for frying.

I've never been massively fond of my veg, but there's no denying that their nutrient and calorie benefits per portion are huge. If you're struggling to eat as much veg as you should, try blending them up into a soup. Add half a tin of chick peas or other beans and you have a low-cal lunch that will see you through the afternoon.

Binge busting

There will be those occasions when you think *To hell with it* and start fantasising about devouring a family pack of crisps or tucking into your favourite pudding. Forearmed is forewarned, so have plenty of fruit on hand as an alternative and keep some yogurt and fruit lollies in the freezer. A can of diet cola can sometimes satisfy those with a sweet tooth and you could hide away a small bar of chocolate for this type of emergency (but only for a real emergency). Popcorn is also a great option as long as you control the portion size (I even developed the MacCorns Binge Buster popcorn for exactly those moments).

20. What works for me

If you want to eat healthily, fat tends to be seen as a dirty word, but things are changing. Could it be the key to losing weight and boosting your brain power? I was interested in the keto diet, so I gave it a try.

For years the 40-40-20 split of carbs-protein-fat has been pretty much accepted among dieticians as a basic structure around which to plan consumption. It's a ratio that I have followed pretty religiously because it provided for the energy, recovery and nutrient demands of my body. That is until recently, when I switched to a diet made up of – wait for it – 75% fat!

This focus on fat is part of a ketogenic diet and it changes the body's primary fuel source from sugar (glucose) derived from carbs, to ketones, produced from fat stored in the liver. It requires a very low carb and protein intake with proteins accounting for around 15% of energy requirements and carbs restricted to 10% at most.

Losing weight, of course, relies on creating a calorie deficit. On a 2000-calorie daily intake that can mean less than 50 grams (one-and-three quarter ounces) of carbs (a baked potato) and 75 grams (two-and-a-half

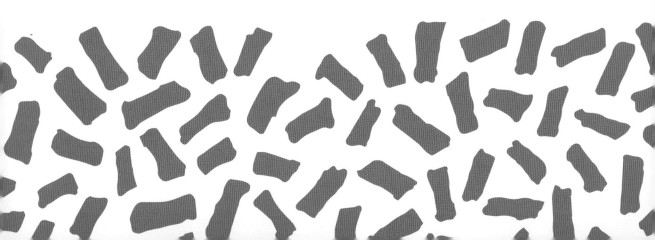

ounces) of protein (a large chicken breast). Instead, on a keto diet, you fill up on fat-heavy foods. These can be the healthy unsaturated fats you find in nuts, seeds, avocados, tofu and olive oil, but also the saturated fats you find in meat, fish, eggs and dairy products, including butter and cream!

Hunger down, energy up

It seems daunting at first. I'd always been reluctant to take the plunge because I love my carbs and still felt they were the only cure for hunger, so I had to adjust my expectations and adjust my meals. Now I typically have eggs for breakfast, a salad with some chicken or fish at lunch and, for supper, meat with plenty of low-carb vegetables such as mushrooms, broccoli, cauliflower or spinach. It's plenty enough to keep me going, and I can honestly say that my appetite and hunger levels have plummeted.

What's more, my energy levels have gone through the roof. I feel supercharged, more than I can ever remember, and it's a feeling that lasts all day. It makes me think that using fat as fuel is similar to putting coals on a fire to keep it going – you get a long, consistent heat. Carbs, on the other hand, are like throwing wood on – the flames flare up for a short period and then die back.

Success with keto relies on bringing your metabolism to what they call 'a state of ketosis' where the body switches from using glucose to ketones. This takes a little patience, as the change can take a few days or even longer. Also, the ratio of carbs necessary to produce ketones varies from person to person and some people will need to reduce their carb intake to as low as 5%. Once you do this, though, weight loss kicks in and it's really not difficult to lose one or two pounds a week.

Lively mind

But there's something else. Once I changed to a keto diet, I found I had more mental focus and greater clarity. I'd read how this could happen, but I wasn't expecting to feel the change. Although not conclusive, there's plenty of scientific research to suggest that the brain, like the rest of the body, derives its energy from glucose and that when forced to use ketones it finds the process more efficient and effective.

This works for me, but switching to a ketogenic diet may not be the best thing for you. There are some possible downsides and if you have liver or kidney problems it could be dangerous. However, my experience has been a positive one. It's had a great effect on both my mind and my body, and I certainly think it's worth looking into further and seeing whether you could benefit.

FOOD AND ME

There was always good food in the house when I was growing up. My dad is part-Italian and my mum's family came from Burma and Asia, so sauces, spices and a variety of tastes were part of my everyday experience. Dining together and enjoying our meals was an important part of our family life. What and how much we ate was never really an issue, and I grew up with a carefree attitude to eating. In fact, my dad and I would sometimes get through a whole loaf of bread at dinner time.

I began to put on weight around the age of 11 and within a few years had noticeably filled out. It was no longer a case of carrying a little puppy fat, but what would now be called obese. I became incredibly self-conscious about it. I would ask my mum to write letters saying I had a cold and couldn't go swimming so I didn't have to undress in front of my classmates, and on holiday I would keep my T-shirt on at the beach even in a heatwave.

And I was bullied. It was mainly name-calling, especially jibes comparing me to a very overweight lad who was a few years ahead of me. I remember looking at him and thinking, 'But I don't look as fat as him, do I?' It was making me unhappy and that had knock-on effects. I lost much of my self-confidence and was becoming withdrawn.

I realise now I was a borderline depressive and hate to think what might have happened had my mum not stepped in. She decided enough was enough and, having introduced me to her friends at the gym, she forced me to get up early and work out before going to school. For a while it was a drag, but with her help I carried on. After a while, it was no longer a chore, but became something I enjoyed. I was losing weight and my body was changing shape without my really noticing.

It was amazing how my self-confidence came back as I lost weight. I began to take pride in how I looked, and was cheerful and chatty. I was also now strong enough to look after not only myself but also other kids who were being bullied. I knew what it felt like and was happy to take on the bullies on their behalf. I got angry at their callousness, but often it ended up in a fight and I'd soon be called to the head's office.

IT WAS NO LONGER A CASE OF CARRYING A LITTLE PUPPY FAT, BUT WHAT THEY WOULD NOW CALL OBESE. I BECAME INCREDIBLY SELF-CONSCIOUS ABOUT IT.

Fast-forward two years. I'm 17 and preparing for my first trip to Ayia Napa with the boys. I was determined to look my best and get myself a proper six-pack before I went. Now, I was a qualified fitness instructor by this point, but had little knowledge of nutrition. I went to the senior bodybuilder in the gym for advice. He told me to stick to a 600-calories-a-day diet. Now, I've got iron willpower and I stuck to it for three months! Never mind that I was killing myself and losing muscle mass, I was building an impressive six-pack and that was the goal.

When I got on the beach at Ayia Napa, my abs were rock hard. There was no way I was going to take it easy on the food and drink out there – I deserved a total blowout – but I really wasn't ready for what happened next. Three months' suffering went down the pan. In just two days, my washboard abs all but disappeared!

I swore I'd never to go such extremes again. I knew there had to be an easier way of getting in trim and not losing it in an instant. And there was. Once I understood more about the way our bodies use food and drink, I realised it's madness to starve yourself. And yet, 9 out of 10 people I train are not eating enough. Their bodies shut down, attempting to conserve energy, and they wonder why they aren't losing weight. When I tell them to eat more to lose weight, they're scared to do it. I'll even tell them I'll pay them if I'm wrong – and I haven't paid out yet!

Ever since then I've managed to keep my weight on an even keel. I eat sensibly and keep my eyes on the scales. Leading such an active life, working with weights most days and training others through the week, means I can eat around 3000 calories a day. That's plenty, even for someone who gets as hungry as I do, and I still don't put on weight. I do, however, still like to get shredded when my body is going to be on display – and I do love to feel the sun on my body when I'm on holiday. After that Ayia Napa disaster, I worked out a 12-week routine that would leave me looking ripped without having to fast. I take it nice and easy, slowly increasing my cardio and decreasing my calories. This was my preparation for going on *Love Island* and by timing it right I managed to look my best when I was on the show.

> **MY PERSONAL DIETING HISTORY HAS MADE ME AWARE OF THE DIFFICULTIES OF LOSING WEIGHT AND I APPRECIATE THE SACRIFICES THAT HAVE TO BE MADE.**

After *Love Island*, however, my life went mad. I was making appearances all around the country and I found it impossible to keep up my routines. Add on the Christmas effect and in six months I had put on a stone since I had been on the show. It wasn't that noticeable to those I met or who saw my photos, but I had been bulking and didn't like it. As 2020 began, I set myself a challenge to get lean and stay like that. This time I gave myself just eight weeks to reach my target weight. That meant dropping my daily calorie allowance by 200 calories each week and adding another five minutes to my cardio as the week went by. By Week 6, I was starting to struggle and Week 7 was pretty tough, but I knew I could get through the last seven days even if the weather closed in and I had to fight my way to the gym through freezing blizzards.

My personal dieting history has made me aware of the difficulties of losing weight and I appreciate the sacrifices that have to be made. On the flipside though, I understand what can be achieved and just what a difference it can make in terms of how you feel within yourself. Helping people improve their health and fitness might be my job, but the satisfaction I get from seeing them succeed is rooted in the fact that I've been there and done that – and I know just how fabulous it feels.

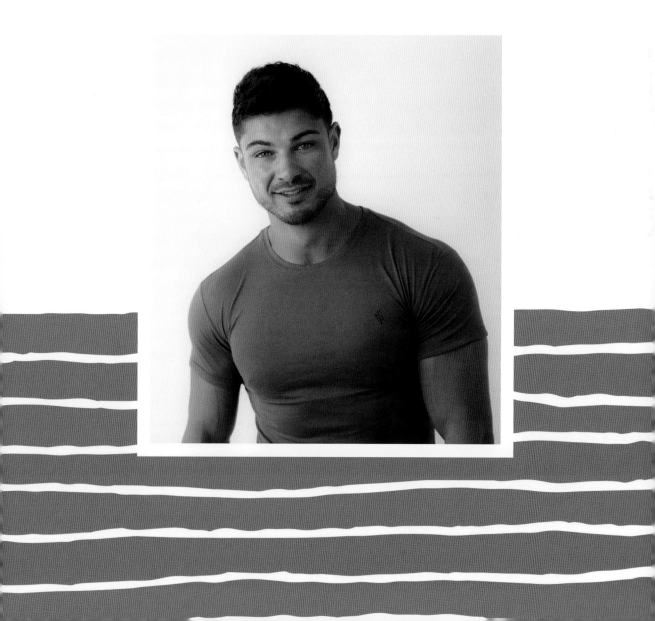

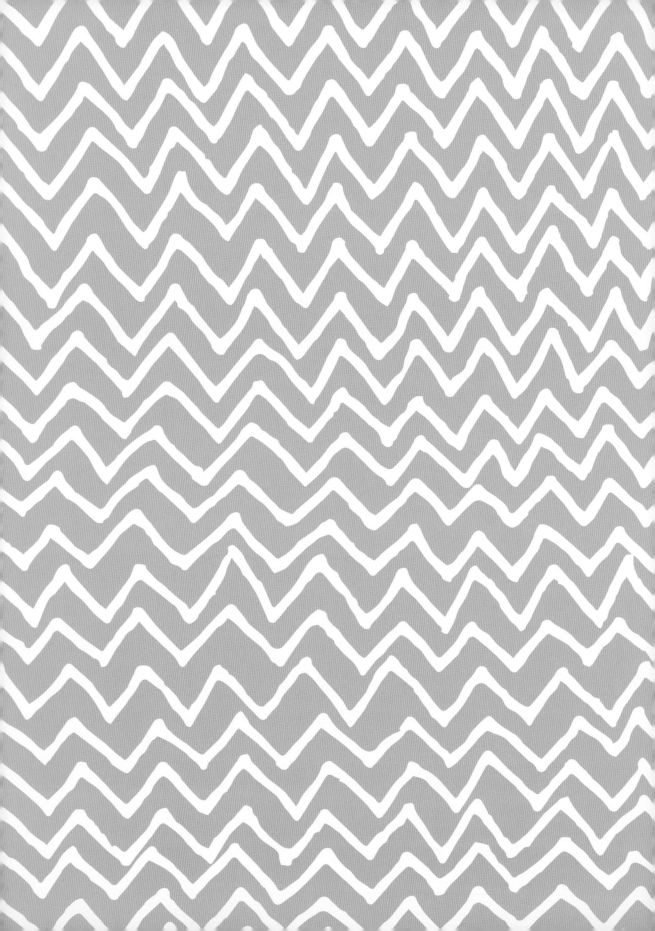

Work

Whether you work for someone else or are building
your own business, career success depends on applying
yourself, dealing with the setbacks and seizing the
opportunities, but don't forget to enjoy it all as well.

21. Develop a work ethic

Without boasting, I like to think I've been pretty successful in my chosen fields, but that's because, although I definitely know how to have a good time, I'm certainly not afraid of hard work either.

After they got married, Mum and Dad decided to set up their own business selling American-style fast food – hamburgers, hot dogs and popcorn. When they set about searching for a popcorn supplier, they had to go all the way to England to find one. Like all sharp entrepreneurs they recognised the gap in the market. So began the story of MacCorns, which is now one of the UK's leading popcorn manufacturers.

That story is one of struggle, graft and grasping opportunity when it arose. Growing up and watching the business develop, it inspired me to become the person I am. When I was five years old, their company had become successful enough to enable them to move to a 30-acre farm in a rural area of Scotland. It was pretty isolated. There weren't gangs of kids around or streets for me to roam. I spent a lot of time with my family and their influence over me was massive – and I'm eternally grateful.

You've got to earn it

I discovered just what a work ethic is through watching them and I understood that you get only what you are prepared to work for. They practised what they preached. I got nothing for nothing. Whereas many of my schoolmates looked forward to a long summer of fun, I knew my days would be spent packing popcorn in the factory. When I asked for a PlayStation, my mum worked out how many hours I'd need to work before they bought me one. I wasn't very happy about it at the time, but I can recognise now the values they were instilling in me.

When I was 17, I began working as a personal trainer and it was those values that drove me to focus single-mindedly on making a success of my career. I'm sure my mum and dad would have found me a place in the family business (and made me work hard at it!), but I knew I had to do something for myself. I'd be up every morning at 5.30am and work through to the evening. I missed out on so much of the fun that many of my mates were having. I gave up football (I wasn't bad – maybe I'd be playing for Scotland by now!) and other sports I loved, and turned down countless nights out with the boys. When I wasn't training, I'd spend every possible minute coming up with ideas to get new clients or delivering leaflets promoting my services.

And you can always do better

When I was 18 or so and beginning to earn decent money, I'd boast to my mum about how much I was bringing home. 'Come back when you've added a zero to that,' she'd reply, bringing me back to earth. They've always said that no matter how well you do, you can always do better, so I should have expected it. They were never ones to tell me (not to my face, at least!) how proud they were of me and they didn't let me to become complacent.

That hasn't changed! When I left *Love Island*, I spent a few weeks on tour in the UK. It doesn't take long to get used to a luxury lifestyle and I began to wonder whether maybe training wasn't the be-all and end-all of everything. It took just a few days at home to put my feet firmly back on the ground. Leaving my mum to clear up my plate after dinner produced a nuclear reaction that shocked me to my senses, while my dad did the same with some choice words: 'Just remember, you're not a celebrity in this house!'

22. Make your own opportunities

You can count yourself lucky if a golden opportunity just presents itself to you. My experience is that most opportunities are the result of careful planning and hard work, and taking them a matter of self-confidence.

It may seem difficult to keep a positive attitude in these days of unpaid internships, minimum wage jobs and zero hours contracts, but self-belief and motivation go a long way to illuminating paths to success. There is no magic key to opening a career door. It probably won't happen quickly or easily and it will almost certainly take a whole lot of work, but with passion and determination you can succeed, because a desire to do what you love and a willingness to make sacrifices can get you over so many obstacles.

What's your passion?

I found something I enjoyed – physical training – and realised I could make some money using my skills to help others. Doctors, musicians, entrepreneurs – people in almost every walk of life will tell you the same story, so decide what you love and, just as importantly, where your talents lie.

Build around your strengths. You might love pop music but not be musical. However, perhaps you can write, draw or communicate well. In the music business, there are many opportunities, including managing, marketing and design. And remember it's not just about money. This is your one life, so if being creative or caring, working outdoors or being among people is important to you, those are valid choices too.

Have a plan

Change in your life is unlikely to happen without input from you. You need to work out where you want to go and how that could happen. When I was young, I knew I wanted to work in fitness. I wasn't sure exactly where or how, so I immersed myself in that world, looking for options and discovering what experience and qualifications I needed to progress. Find a mentor or someone who can advise you in your field and set yourself some achievable short-term goals that will set you on your way.

Be prepared to change course. You're going to encounter setbacks or even failures, but take the view that they were somehow meant to happen and see them as part of the learning process. You might need to change your level of commitment. You might have to reassess your plan or reconsider your long-term goal. Before *Love Island*, when I failed the audition for a TV show called *Survival of the Fittest*, I took it as a sign. I needed to practise and be more prepared. Don't stand still. Ask yourself the tough questions such as: *Am I on the right road? Is this course of action effective? Is this the best I can do?* And if you answer no, do something about it!

Be adventurous

The real secret of most successful people is that they aren't scared to take a risk. That doesn't mean they're cocky or arrogant; most are just quietly confident of their abilities. Opportunities are like throwing a double in snakes and ladders – a great chance to jump ahead.

At a young age I was given a chance to take a large fitness class when another trainer failed to turn up. I was so nervous, but deep down I knew I could do it. Later, when I was offered a place on *Love Island*, I knew I might end up looking a real prat, but I was confident that the public would see my real personality. You have to be constantly on the lookout for opportunities and you have to work out whether they will help you achieve your goals. If they do, put your nerves, doubts and what-ifs to one side and back yourself to succeed.

23. Build a business

Whether you're building a business or forging a career, your success depends on how much you want it. If you're willing to make sacrifices, take risks, ride every setback and – you can't avoid it – work hard, then go for it!

I like making money. As long as you're treating your employees well and giving value for money to your clients or customers, then I really think you can take pride in it. I suppose it was watching my parents build their business that gave me the entrepreneurial bug. It was certainly something I caught at an early age. One time, when I was at school, my mum and dad were called in to see the headteacher. I'd been taking popcorn in to sell to the other kids and I was making a bomb. I don't think the head would have worried too much, but I was taking more money in than the school tuck shop!

How I did it

When I was 17, I had my first client as a personal trainer. I gave her cheap rates because I was eager to gain experience. After a month, she doubled my money – £10 for every inch she'd cut from her waistline! I was thrilled about her success, but equally excited to earn proper money under my own steam. I loved that feeling of working for myself and bringing in money, and it was a feeling that would inspire me to work even harder in the coming years.

For the next five years I single-mindedly worked to build a fitness business of my own. I sacrificed many of the things people enjoy about being young: friendships, big nights out with mates and holidays, and I relied on girlfriends being understanding. All this is not meant to sound big-headed. Up and down the country, many people are doing the same. Working for yourself is loads of people's ultimate dream: no boss, work any hours you want, pay yourself. That's all true, but there's another side to that coin. You take responsibility for everything; you're the only one who's going to get the work done, even if it takes all day. And if you don't earn money, you don't take money home.

Don't stop learning

For me, and for many setting out to build a business, learning was an everyday experience. I took advice everywhere I could find it. If you're lucky, you might find someone who is happy to mentor you. I talked to senior trainers at the gym and others who were running similar operations. I gleaned whatever I could from them, but I also constantly read magazine articles and books, and watched videos to improve my knowledge. These were not necessarily directly related to training. Sometimes they were about motivation, diet or life coaching, but they gave me a different perspective on what I was trying to achieve.

Making decisions can often be a daunting task when you're inexperienced. Try to understand your strengths and weaknesses. You may be good with people, but awful with figures. You could be great at tech, but lack inspiration for marketing the business. Don't be afraid to ask for advice and to lean on those you know have the skills to help. For years my dad has been great in helping with my accounts and tax returns, and I had a girlfriend who showed me exactly how to use Facebook to promote the business effectively.

I've never regretted setting up in business on my own. It can be a rollercoaster of an adventure, but the freedom, responsibilities and successes are thrilling, and there is no better feeling than earning money through your own initiative, skills and hard work.

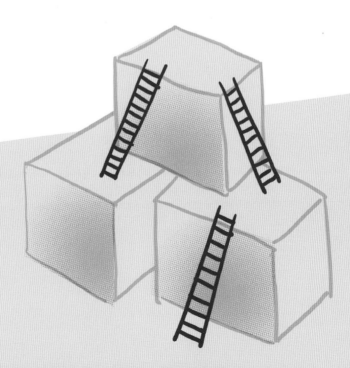

24. Enjoy your success

To be successful you need desire, ambition and hard work. But no matter who you are, if you want to do what you love and love what you do, the opportunities are out there for you...

I've talked about how as a young man I was motivated by money. That was true – the thought of making good money spurred me to work harder and harder. Although I had already discovered that the gym was a place I felt comfortable and fulfilled, I like to think that I would have strived as hard to make it in any other sphere I'd chosen. However, I found out something else about myself which made it even more enjoyable. As much as I liked being paid by my clients, I realised how much satisfaction I was increasingly getting from helping them achieve their goals.

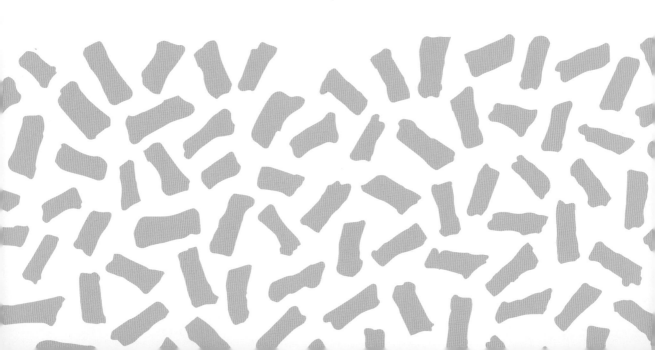

Finding job satisfaction

The thanks and presents from those who had already paid me for guiding them to their weight and fitness targets gave me such a glow. To successfully help someone effect a positive change in their life was an amazing feeling – even better than changing my own. To find something that you are genuinely proud of doing, in whatever field you choose to work, makes it so much more worthwhile.

When I left *Love Island*, so many opportunities suddenly opened up for me. They may have been lucrative and even fun, but I chose to stick with the career I had started. I loved training more than anything and realised that if I used the TV exposure and media spotlight well, it could help me achieve more of my ambitions. One of the main reasons I went on the show was to raise my profile with a young audience. Now I was able to tour schools where the children recognised me and were eager to listen to my message about the importance of fitness.

Enough success to go around

We can't all be CEOs, billionaires, celebrities or sports stars, but we can all recognise success in our own lives. I started as a money-orientated teenager, but as I have grown up I've realised that success is not only measured in money. I've grown to value what I can do for others and how working makes me appreciate the time I spend with my family, friends or just getting away from it all.

My story isn't rags to riches. I was well provided for and my parents really supported me – my mum persuading a boot camp company who wanted to use the Ranch to take me on as an instructor was one of my big breaks. There are plenty of people who have come from far less privileged backgrounds than myself and made a great success of their careers, and they are the role models for us all.

Success is open to everyone. It's something you should never feel resentful or competitive about – others being successful doesn't take away your opportunities. There's plenty enough success in the world for us all, so go and grab your share.

MAKING A CHANGE

Having settled down to my school studies, I assumed I would go on to university once I finished my Highers (Scottish school leaving exams). I had no specific ambitions, but knew I wanted to work in sport and fitness, so I was looking at sports science courses. I am, however, a great believer in taking your chances when they appear and an opportunity arose that I felt I just couldn't turn down.

I'd been working out in the gym ever since I was 15 years old. I was pretty obsessed with it and spent much of my time hanging out there. I knew about form, how to use weights and which muscles I was focusing on, but wasn't that clued up on much of the science. Then, when I was 17, a fitness company approached my parents to ask to use the Ranch facilities in order to run a boot camp. As part of the deal, my mum, always looking for a chance to help me get on, asked if they would take me on to help with the training.

I threw myself into it. I watched carefully how and what the instructors communicated, and made myself as useful as I possibly could. Soon I was working regularly with the company and loving every moment of it. When it came to leaving school, I knew I wasn't going to take up the place I had to study at uni; from now on my education was going to be on the job.

It can be scary when you're thrown in at the deep end, but sometimes that sink or swim moment can prove to be the best way of taking a step forward. One day, when I was meant to be assisting a trainer with his class at the Ranch, I received a last-minute text saying he wasn't able to make it and I would have to cover for him. I was so nervous. I had never taken a class before and didn't believe I was ready. However, it went really well and that gave me so much confidence. I was an instructor now and was hungry for more!

I talked to experienced trainers, immersed myself in books, learned about nutrition and how the body works, and studied for my qualifications. I even began taking on personal clients of my own. I started out by training two people in the field by the Ranch. It felt great to earn my own money doing something I absolutely loved. I got a real buzz from helping people feel better and I seemed to be good at it. People responded to my character and the positive message I was putting out. As more people signed up, my life became training people, keeping myself fit and toned, and learning to run my own business.

WHEN IT CAME TO LEAVING SCHOOL, I KNEW I WASN'T GOING TO TAKE UP THE PLACE I HAD TO STUDY AT UNI; FROM NOW ON MY EDUCATION WAS GOING TO BE ON THE JOB.

It took up all my time. By now my long-term girlfriend had gone off to uni and pretty soon that led to us going our separate ways. Although it was a mutual decision, it was still a great wrench, but fortunately I had my work to keep me from reflecting on it too much. I was so engrossed in training and working that any thoughts of serious relationships were put aside for the time being. It wasn't that I never went out or saw friends, but I was motivated by getting the business going and I would nearly always prioritise that over socialising.

Just 18 months after starting out, I was training 50 people and running three or four boot camps a week. All this had been taking place outdoors on the Ranch, but I knew if I was going to develop my business I'd need some indoor space. On the property there was an old woodshed that I realised I could use. I cleared the wood out and set about transforming it in to my own gym. At the beginning there was just some very basic equipment and a few mats, but it was enough for me to take classes there. When I could I'd invest in new machines, improving the facilities all the time.

I WAS SO COMMITTED TO MAKING THE BUSINESS WORK. I'D BE IN THE GYM AT 6.30AM AND WOULDN'T LOCK UP UNTIL 9PM. WHEN I WASN'T WORKING OUT MYSELF OR TRAINING OTHERS, I'D BE COMING UP WITH IDEAS TO GET NEW CLIENTS AND HANDING OUT LEAFLETS IN THE LOCAL TOWNS.

I was so committed to making the business work. I'd be in the gym at 6.30am and wouldn't lock up until 9pm. When I wasn't working out myself or training others, I'd be coming up with ideas to get new clients and handing out leaflets in the local towns. Suddenly I was making decent money, especially compared to my friends who were still at uni.

I now had my own place to live, but I hadn't gone far. As a 19-year-old, I had been looking to move out of the family home and get my own space. It was my mum's idea that I take the chalet which they had built on the grounds of the Ranch. They built it after my gran died so that my grandad could live nearby but still have his own independence. However, when it came to it, he couldn't face leaving his friends and the neighbourhood he had lived in for so long, but I jumped at the chance to move in.

I could now invite my friends and girlfriends over without disturbing anyone and have some privacy whenever I wanted. It did feel a little odd, though. All my life I'd always been so close to my family and although they were just a couple of minutes away, it seemed, well, different. My mum clearly thought the same thing. It was a matter of days before she told me she was missing me and asked if I'd come back for dinner every night.

When I left school, I would never have guessed how the next few years would pan out. I can see now a combination of hard work, taking the opportunities that came my way and having a passion for what I did helped me carve out a good lifestyle for myself. I still had a lot to learn, but I knew that fitness was an area which I loved working in, that helping people feel better about themselves made me feel good too, and that running a successful business was something I could do pretty well. I was well set.

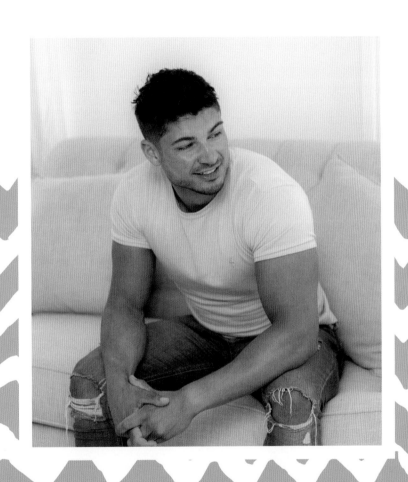

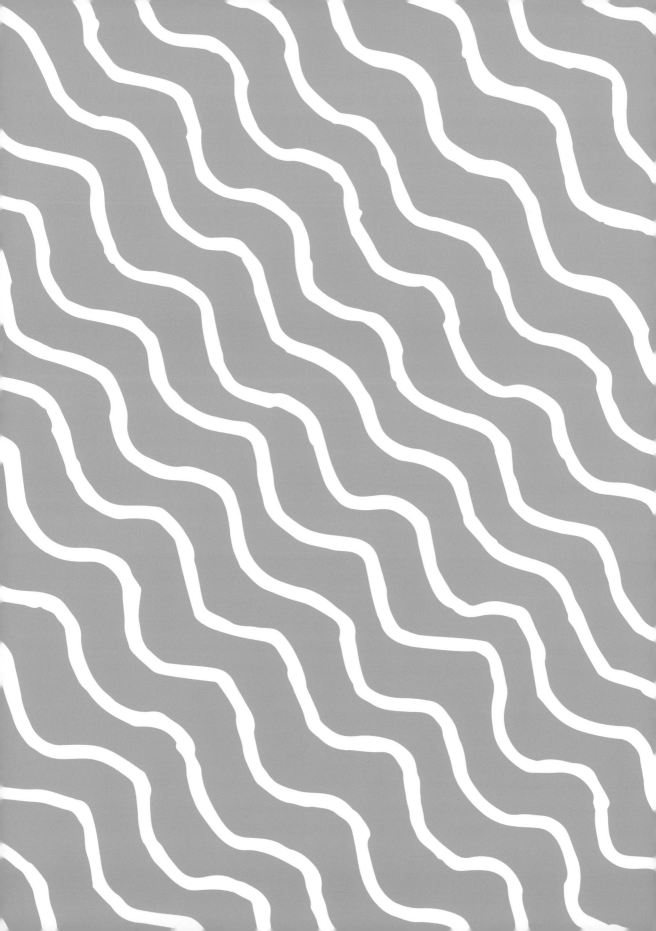

Relationships

There's nothing like your first love. You want it to last forever. It's a totally consuming feeling. But relationships can be tricky. How do you deal with disagreements? How do you let go? And is hanging on ultimately worse?

25. First love

Look, I can't claim to be the world's greatest expert, but I do have some romantic experience and I know what the joy and the pain of first love are like.

I met my first love when I was 15. She was in the year below at school and it seemed like we were made for each other. We'd spend every moment we could together – kissing and cuddling at lunchtimes, meeting after school, doing homework together. For two years we were inseparable and I couldn't imagine being without her.

We didn't believe the end of our schooldays would change anything. Sure, she was going to university and I was staying behind to work as a trainer, but we wouldn't be far apart. It didn't take long to realise we were wrong. We had different lifestyles. She was enjoying the student social life to the full and I was working seven days a week. As much as we still loved each other, it was just unworkable. Both in floods of tears, we agreed to split up and go our separate ways. We didn't even stay in contact.

You don't forget

That experience of first love is still vividly imprinted on my mind (or, for the more romantically inclined, on my heart). The emotions I felt were new and intense. I had desired and loved and found those feelings reciprocated in the purest form I could imagine. I immediately started seeing someone else and desperately tried to find those same levels of passion. After six months I gave up and returned to my first love. We stayed together for a year, but the magic had gone; our lives had moved in different directions. I finished the relationship just before Valentine's Day. I could tell she was upset, but she had so much self-respect and just calmly walked away.

Rekindling a first-love relationship, trying to replicate those intense emotions in subsequent relationships, even wanting that same feeling of heartbreak when you split up – they are all classic traps and I fell into them. They can also be harmful for your future romantic prospects. The key is in the word 'first'. The euphoric feelings you get from that initial relationship may seem stronger and more powerful because that was the first time you experienced them – even more if they are magnified by teenage hormones and brain development. So maybe the first – and harshest – lesson is that you'll never feel that way again, so get over it!

But don't live in the past

It's so easy to see that first love with a rose-tinted glow. Was it really all good? Was it sustainable into adulthood? How dependent was it on being responsibility-free young souls? I wouldn't recommend it as a strategy, but getting back with my first love showed me that, ultimately, we weren't as compatible as I once imagined and that helped me move on.

The next step takes some discipline. Live in the present. Accept that you experienced something wonderful, but also accept that it was in the past and you were both different people then. Don't let yourself be imprisoned by your own memories when there are so many new experiences and encounters open to you. Your new relationships will have their own characteristics and emotions, and they don't need to be continually compared to some idealised love.

You'll probably never forget that first love, but you can lock those recollections away in the back of your mind where they won't cause harm. One day you can dig them out and enjoy them for what they were: golden memories of a love that could only have happened in those innocent days of your youth.

26. Significant others

Is he or she a keeper? Long-term relationships can be a source of great contentment and security, but also of conflict and unhappiness. Getting it right is one of the most important issues in life.

Having a stable, happy relationship is such an important part of life. Although some people are perfectly content to live a single life, and I'm one of them at the moment, sharing love, companionship and a physical relationship with a partner is something that can bring out the best in you.

My time on *Love Island* made me realise that it's so easy to fall for someone if you can enjoy a lot of time with them away from it all. It's artificial, though, as Belle and I discovered. When you have to cope with the hassles and distractions of everyday life, if you're both going to feel nourished by it, a relationship needs to be solid in so many areas.

Appearances matter

Yes, looks do matter. I'd be crazy to say otherwise. It provides the initial spark that draws you to someone, and physical attraction continues to be a vital part of a relationship. It's just a part, though and you need to make other connections. The problem can be that the physical magnetism is initially so strong that it overshadows other considerations; issues that can sooner or later lead to you being very unfulfilled and unhappy.

We all try to present our best selves at the start of a relationship. It's only natural. We want to impress. Trying to be someone you aren't, though, is only going to cause problems later. You are who you are and if they don't like that, they never will. You shouldn't have to change for them and, just as importantly, you have no right to demand that they change for you.

What's important

If you can't live with their different approach to whatever it is that's important to you – time together, money, politics – it's better not to start. I'm a regimented person who loves routine. I now know to end a developing relationship when someone has a more carefree, perhaps chaotic attitude to life. They're not wrong and I don't believe I am either – I just can't see it working out.

No relationship is going to be perfect. It's all about how much you're both willing to compromise; how much you want to give to and take from each other. When it works it's the greatest thing, even if it doesn't last forever. But it can. I only have to look at my parents to know that. I'm not claiming to be an expert, but from observing their relationship and from my own experience, there are certain things which are key…

Making it work

Stay honest: An open and true conversation is what bonds two people together. Without that you don't have a relationship.

Be best friends: Share the good times and the bad. Help each another attain your goals by being a sounding board, a mentor, a shoulder to cry on or just someone it's easy to spend time with.

Be emotionally mature: There will be testing times in any relationship when you need to dig deep and be willing to listen, compromise and even forgive.

Add to each other's life: If you let it, every relationship has a capacity to mutually enhance each other's lives with humour and empathy, as well as new perspectives, new experiences and new people.

Do nothing: Great couples can be comfortable with each other without doing anything. When you don't need to interact, talk or do things together, but still feel the love, then I think you have truly cracked it.

27. Learn to argue

All couples argue. In fact, if you're not prepared to give your opinion, then it might be a sign that all isn't well in the relationship. However, it's so easy for the ways in which we argue to be destructive and even hurtful.

Years before *Love Island*, I took part in an internet reality show called *Glow*, a Glasgow version of *TOWIE*. Towards the end of my time on the show, the cameras caught what I believed to be a private argument I was having with my then girlfriend, Denise. I certainly wouldn't have argued like that if I knew I was being filmed and I received a barrage of online abuse for how I acted. However, watching it back, I was shocked at my behaviour, particularly the aggression I showed towards someone for whom I felt genuine affection.

I'm an emotional person and am quick to take issue with any criticism I see as unfair. Some might say I take slights too personally. I've made a conscious effort to be calm and measured in any arguments I get into, and here are a few of the points I try to follow…

- **Stay humble:** Don't assume the moral high ground. Not only is it condescending and can escalate ill feeling, but there's a chance you're in for a shock. Be prepared to be proven wrong.

- **Think before you speak:** It's tempting to reel off every opinion as it comes into your head, but pause and sift through them. Do they make a fair point and move the argument on? If they're irrelevant, insulting or petty, then put them on one side.

- **Don't get personal:** Arguments are no time to be deliberately hurtful, so don't make remarks about personal features or family members. Similarly, bringing up sore points from the past and issues that have been dealt with in previous discussions will only make matters worse.

- **Listen:** Give the person you're arguing with a fair chance to speak without interruption and actually listen to them. Acknowledge what they are saying even if you don't agree. Try arguing as if you're right, but listening as if you're wrong.

- **Curb your aggression:** Begin with 'I' and not 'you'. Better still, try 'I feel…' because it's less confrontational. Shouting louder doesn't make you any more right. Try lowering your voice instead if you're trying to insist on a point. And, there is never, ever a reason to use physical force. If you feel either of you are losing control, suggest time out – a short break in which you can calm down.

- **Your relationship is worth more than winning an argument:** Always bear in mind how much this friendship and relationship means to you. If you want to keep it, then stay civil, don't let it escalate and remind them that this is just one small issue among the many things you love about them. Don't throw the baby out with the bathwater.

That *Love Island* row

Hopefully those who watched my (the world's most disastrous) proposal to Belle on *Love Island* will see I've made some progress (even if they thought I was in the wrong). When Belle ripped into me over kissing Anna in the 'Snog, Marry, Pie' game, I tried not to react emotionally and to have a calm discussion. I ended up walking away rather than inflaming the situation further. It's not easy to keep a cool head when your integrity and character are questioned, but in the long run it does pay dividends. We were able to make up quickly and even become close enough to see each other when we left the island.

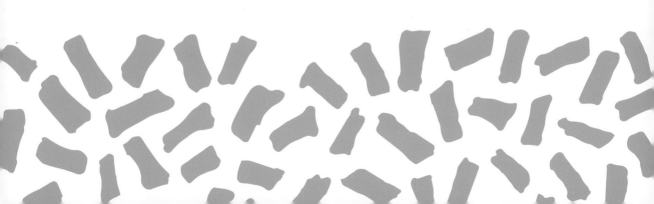

TAKING A CHANCE

You wouldn't think this was the case if you read the tabloids who just love to build me up as a party animal, a lothario or a love rat, but I think of my life between 18 and going on *Love Island* as being a time when I worked hard to develop the business, spent time with my family and enjoyed quiet nights in with the steady girlfriends I had in those years. To be perfectly honest, the majority of my time was spent in the gym – possibly to the detriment of those relationships. I loved the workouts, chatting to the members who used it and working with the people I was training.

I was a pretty normal young man. I did socialise with my friends whether it was in a bar, on holiday or just watching a film at home, but I didn't really drink much and wouldn't touch drugs – there was no point being so committed to my training and wrecking it with that kind of thing. That said, I can't deny having the odd raucous night out with the boys and the occasional clubbing and beach break in Ibiza – and, no shock here, there were girls around.

I was, and still am, proud of my looks. I'd scrub up well, had a good body and was well aware that I could make an impression. I enjoyed the attention and sometimes couldn't resist taking things further with some of the girls I chatted with. Now I deeply regret the hurt I caused by two-timing my girlfriends, but at the time I was young and believed I was just having some fun.

The whole 'my mum shaves my bum' story goes back to this time too. When I was 18 I was offered the chance to earn some extra money by appearing at parties as a 'Butler in the Buff'. Of course, I cringe now at the idea, but at the time it was easy money and a lot of fun. I wasn't totally naked, as I had a posing pouch to cover my modesty. This did, however, expose my backside, which I knew was quite hairy, so it seemed natural to ask my mum to shave it. What else was I supposed to do?

My first instinct to any offer is to say 'yes'. I love the idea of taking on new challenges, and that attitude has served me pretty well over the years. Perhaps the one exception is *Glow*. In 2016 *Glow* was launched as Glasgow's version of *The Only Way is Essex*, even if it was only broadcast online. The idea was to present the day-to-day life of the city's 'beautiful people' and the producers had high hopes that it would be taken up by a TV channel. I was 21 and getting on with my fitness work. I really wasn't looking to be in a reality show and they didn't come looking for me, but I ended up on the show.

When I split with my first girlfriend, I went to Ibiza with some friends. Although some might advise against starting a relationship on the rebound, I met Denise and we carried on seeing each other when we got back from the holiday. She had already been selected to be a major cast member of *Glow* and, as her boyfriend, I was invited to join them. Always up for anything, I said yes, but fairly soon I was regretting the once- or twice-weekly filming, and the show wasn't all it promised to be. There was little about it that was 'classy' and instead it focused on bust-ups and fights. Denise and I had already split up when they staged an explosive argument in which she accused me of cheating on her. The series never made it on to TV, but it was quite popular in Scotland. I didn't enjoy the experience, but I learned some useful lessons about how I came across on screen, and it gave me a taste of what it was like being in the spotlight.

To be honest, it was a relief to get back to the Ranch and focus on my work. Among my clients there were a few younger kids who had been brought along by their parents, and working with them was really rewarding. I was still quite young myself and I think they found they could relate to me, my sense of humour and what I was putting across. Perhaps they were even inspired by me! When

I was 21, I started running summer camps focussing on fitness for kids aged between five and 12. We'd have great fun with the exercises, and I'd teach them about healthy eating and keeping themselves fit. The kids loved it and I got great feedback from the parents who told me how much the youngsters got out of it.

I remembered the mental and physical benefits I received through learning to get fit and look after my body when I was young. I knew just what a transformation that feeling can make to a person's self-esteem, especially at such an emotionally vulnerable time as childhood and the teenage years, and studies show that kids who enjoy sport and exercise at that age tend to stay active throughout their lives. I was in my element and decided this was where I wanted to focus my energies in the future.

By this point the gym was fully furnished and flourishing. I had 300 members and was employing quite a few staff, so with less pressure on my time I was able to focus on kids' fitness. I looked for other opportunities to communicate with them and at that time apps were gaining traction, but DVDs were still pretty popular, so I decided to make a kids' fitness DVD. However, the next problem was that I was only known in the local area and by those in Scotland who had watched *Glow* – hardly a mass audience and nowhere near the right demographic!

Looking at the steps other people have taken often gives you clues as to how you might emulate their achievements. At that time Charlotte Crosby's *3 Minute Belly Blitz* was the UK's biggest selling fitness DVD. Charlotte had first gained fame on *Geordie Shore*, the reality series set in Newcastle-upon-Tyne, and had used her celebrity status to promote the DVD to great effect. My first stop had to be her agents, Bold Management, to see if they could help me launch my kids' DVD.

They explained that without a public profile to speak of there was little they could do for me. Now I'm not one to take 'no' for an answer, but my mum, she takes it personally. She rang them up and, trying not to shout, said, 'Listen, have you seen my ****ing boy?' She sent a set of my photos and within 10 minutes they called back, telling her they'd be happy to try to place me on a reality show! I was up for that. I'd learned from my time on *Glow* and was confident that, given a chance, I could make a favourable impression with TV audiences.

Bold were true to their word. They got me an audition for a new reality show called *Survival of the Fittest*. Capitalising on the success of the first series of *Love Island*, this series was planned as a winter 'sister' series. Teams of six girls and boys would live together in a South African lodge and compete against each other in mental and physical challenges. The show also had a dating element and all the contestants were single. OK, I wasn't actually single when I went up for the show, but I figured I'd cross that bridge when the time came.

I needn't have worried. I never reached that bridge. I did the worst audition ever! I can't blame the producers for rejecting me. I like to think that everything happens for a reason, and the only thing I could do was learn from my mistakes. I swore that next time I'd be better prepared. *Love Island* was made by the same production company as *Survival of the Fittest* and I was soon asked to attend an audition for that series. I suppose they must have seen something in me despite my awful first impression. I was conflicted. I was still eager to raise my profile and make the DVD, but by now I was in a serious relationship – one I didn't want to end, lie about or jeopardise by flirting with other girls in front of millions. I turned down the opportunity.

Love Island went from strength to strength. The introduction of Casa Amor – the luxury bolthole where contestants are tempted by new arrivals – just added to the show's popularity. The 2018 series (won by Dani Dyer and Jack Fincham) was the most popular so far: around four million people watched each episode. I was one of them. I liked the setting, the drama, the laughs and the good-looking girls and guys – and, maybe just occasionally, I let myself imagine how I might get on if I ever got to enter the villa…

Dealing with stress

Every life comes with its own worries, stresses and strains. Some can be ignored, others need to be faced. Fortunately, there are strategies and techniques which can prevent them from weighing you down.

28. Feeling blue

We all get down. It can be over something genuinely upsetting, something trivial or for no apparent reason at all. We may not be able to completely control our negative thoughts, but we can train ourselves to recognise the onset of the 'blues' and find coping mechanisms that help.

Getting knocked back by the girls in front of the millions watching *Love Island* wasn't easy. It did hit me hard, but I knew I had two choices. I could react by sulking and being miserable or I could see the funny side and bounce back. I knew I was strong enough to laugh at myself, and had the confidence and character to pull it off. I also know that not everyone would have felt the same, so focus on who you are and where your inner strength comes from.

We only really have two kinds of thoughts: positive and negative. According to some scientists we have at least 60,000 thoughts day, so it stands to reason that some of them (some claim 80% of them!) are going to be negative. It's not just you. Celebrities, vloggers, musicians are no different – they all get down too. It's just some of them are better at dealing with it than others. Bad and sad things are going to happen to us all and sometimes we feel low for no reason, but accepting that you're not going to feel totally upbeat 24/7 is the first step in dealing with it.

Settle on a routine

If you have a routine in your life, stick to it. It'll help you get through the day and move your mind on. I do cardio exercises in the morning – every morning. I don't have to think about it and as soon as I'm into it my mind is occupied. Plan your day and stick to it. That doesn't mean you can't spend time mulling things over in your head if you need to, but allocate some time to it and move on when the time is up.

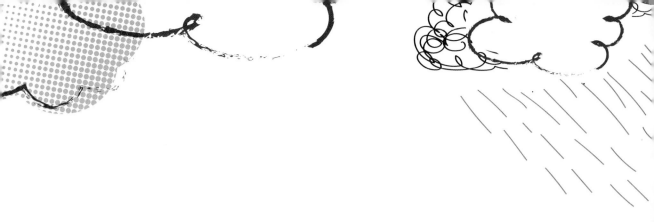

Just as working out helps your body become stronger, you can train your mind to seek out the positive. Recognise when and why you're feeling good about life. Store that thought and apply that way of thinking when other things happen. For example, if you find yourself reflecting on a good time spent with friends, work out what it was you enjoyed and link it to other occasions when you felt like that. You can build a kind of library of positive thoughts in your head, which you can dip into whenever you need. Just as you might challenge yourself in the gym, force yourself to find the positive in increasingly tough scenarios until it becomes second nature.

Have a reaction plan

Be prepared for the times when those grey clouds arrive – because sooner or later, they will. We all have something we can use as a mood changer. Personally, I go back to the gym. A solid session, sometimes listening to a positivity podcast – like a lot of other people, I like Paul McKenna's – changes my mindset. For other people it might be playing an instrument, listening to certain music, watching a favourite movie or spending time with your pet. Helping someone, reading, walking – whatever it is, immerse yourself in the activity and you'll find it improves your outlook and refreshes your mood.

It's really important to assess what's causing your negativity. If it's out of your control – anything from a friend moving away to your team's defeat – accept that and concentrate on turning round your reaction. However, pain can also be a catalyst for change. It can provide the push you need to improve a situation and feel better about yourself. Perhaps you could alter how you behave, maybe get yourself fit or look for a new job? What I do know is that making your blue moods work for you and changing a negative thought to a positive action is one of the best feelings ever.

29. Don't stress yourself

Stress is just part of life, but unless we manage our anxiety it can stop us getting on with what's important, disrupt our relationships and even affect our physical wellbeing.

I'd describe myself as quite emotional, a bit of a control freak and an overthinker. I still find myself debating whether to put the tea or milk in the cup first – which is prime stress material for you. I can get infuriated with work when things don't go well and I become frustrated with people for a host of reasons. Imagine how I felt, then, in the early weeks on *Love Island*, when there were cameras everywhere, new people to not only meet but live with, and millions watching. I can honestly say those were some of the most stressful times I've ever experienced!

There's a saying I love, 'The same boiling water which softens the potato also hardens the egg.' That's to say, it's not the circumstances that create the stress, but the make-up of the person. During my time in the villa, I tried to be as egg-like as I could. Before I started, the production team told me to savour the time on the programme. Those words were always in my mind when things got tough, because I knew they were right and I knew that worrying about what people at home were saying would ruin the whole amazing experience.

Can you control it?

The key to dealing with stress is to assess what you can and cannot control. There are many things you can't stop from happening, from a bus strike to a heatwave. What you can control is your own reaction to these things. You can think about how you will get to work or what preparations you might make for extreme weather. You can't do anything about the bad behaviour of a friend or relative, but you have total power over how you choose to react.

Of course, problems arise; they always will. However, you can learn to deal with them in a calm way. For every worry you have, there should be only two options: do something or change your thinking. Think practically about what action you need to take, and when and how you will go about it. If you can't make a plan, then focus on your emotional state. Are you worrying unnecessarily about something beyond your control, something that you can deal with when or if it happens or something trivial that really isn't a problem at all? Take time to clear your head, rationalise your thoughts and manage your stress.

Some stress-control tips

Get physical: Exercise is a top stress-reliever. The focus and repetitive actions relax the mind, much like meditation. It can reduce tension and anxiety and may release endorphins, the brain's feel-good signals.

Sleep, sleep, sleep: Sleeping can help restore many of the body's functions that are put under pressure by stress and anxiety. Sticking to a regular sleep routine can help improve your mood, concentration and problem solving.

Stay positive: Have faith in your own decision-making and trust the process. If you've thought a situation through, then things usually work out. If not, you'll be able to adapt and find another solution.

Give yourself worry time: It's natural to be anxious about all kinds of things – but not all the time. If it helps, allocate yourself some time to worry and then switch off – watch TV, go for a run, call a friend – when the time is up.

Get some advice: Some people just seem to soak up any stress, at least on the surface, while others are less good at dealing with it. Sometimes talking through a problem with someone you trust can help, but remember it's not a sign of weakness or inadequacy to feel overwhelmed by stress, and in those situations consider getting some help from a professional – it's definitely not something to feel embarrassed about.

30. Money matters

Money worries are probably one of the most – if not the most – common causes of stress. There are no easy solutions to financial problems, but it is possible to reduce the numbing, all-consuming pain that they can induce.

We all spend far too much time worrying about money. And I'm not just saying that as someone who doesn't have too many financial concerns at the moment, because like most people there have been times when I've wondered just how I'm going to pay the bills. None of us want money worries to affect our lives, so that means we need to find a way to work out how to deal with it, follow the plan and then put those troubling thoughts aside.

Managing money comes easier to some than others. Although my parents went through some tough years as they built their business, I never wanted for anything. When I was 17, my friends and I booked a holiday to Ayia Napa. Down at the travel agent, they all had the money to pay for it there and then, but although I knew I could get my parents to pay for me, I decided to pay it off in instalments – by myself.

Extravagant purchases

Not that I was always so sensible. A couple years later, my business had grown and I felt a need to show everyone how well I was doing. I bought a Mercedes, but had a yearning for a Porsche. I took the plunge despite only just being able to make the payments. When the business subsequently took an unexpected plunge, I became really stressed about how I'd pay for it. Somehow, even if the cash came through on the day the payment was due, I always just made it. 'You're such a lucky bastard,' my mum would say when I told her.

The anxiety caused by money is probably the hardest of all. For many people, it is an ever-present, nagging worry, a dark cloud that follows them around, and at its worst it can have a paralysing effect on your whole life. Like all stressful situations, there are really only two actions you can take: assess your emotional reaction, then make and follow a plan.

Basic budgeting

Working out a budget does require a bit of maths. You need to be honest and clear about your financial situation: how much money you have coming in, what bills you absolutely have to pay, and what debt or savings you might have. Then review your spending patterns. Where does the money go? Are you spending too much time on Amazon, Asos and other online shopping sites? Do you love a shopping spree or a big night out? Is credit card interest taking a big slice? And count the small amounts. A coffee, a trip to the nail bar, a present for a friend, a delivery pizza – they all add up. Only then can you work out what you have to spend, how you'll save for a holiday or special purchase, or pay off your debts.

If you seek advice from a friend, relative or professional, do it calmly and listen to what they say. Make a plan that you can live with. The essentials of food, accommodation and bills must be covered, but it's OK to allow yourself some small indulgences, perhaps a gym membership, an occasional trip to the cinema or even just a coffee with a friend once a week. Once you have the plan, stick to it and review it regularly. Pay rises, changes in interest rates or lifestyle changes can all impact your finances more than you might imagine.

Now get on with your life. Focus on the present. If you start to worry about a pension, paying next year's tax or a car repair bill, put aside time to work out what to do. Don't let the worry fester, and tackle it by thinking through your budget. Ignoring your finances won't help you break the habit of angsting about money, but when you do, you'll find it's liberating.

31. Red mist

Everyone loses their rag now and then. With luck, it's all sorted out in minutes. But angry confrontations can have severe consequences. It's time everyone calmed down...

Anger is an odd thing, isn't it? One person might get angry at politics, another at her boyfriend, another at being stuck in a traffic jam. No two people are alike. Nearly everyone has a trigger, but what they respond to and how severely they react is so individual.

I've got a bad temper. My triggers are usually other people's behaviour, often when they are late or rude (especially on Instagram!). But I can get angry with myself too. Foods affect my moods. If I overeat, I can get so annoyed with myself, and if I'm in the last weeks of a diet, I can be so on edge it's unreal. My mum says she can tell exactly how close I am to losing it just by looking at my face.

Not nice

Unfortunately, the public got to see the worst of me when I was on the *Glow* reality show. I had a stand-up row with Denise and just flipped. It wasn't pretty and I was totally embarrassed that my friends and parents watched it. It's a good guide – if you are looking for ways not to act. I raised my voice, said things I didn't mean and my body language was aggressive. Watching it back taught me a lot about my behaviour. Maybe all our tantrums should be filmed and played back to us later!

Anger is a natural emotion, but we can try to control its effect on ourselves. As I've got older, I've learned to give people a little more leeway and understand that they might be under their own stresses and pressures. I recognise that anger is a wasted energy that I could channel more effectively in other directions, and I realise that it's connected with my own frustrations.

Find a way to vent

As part of my training routine, I've taken up boxing over the last couple of years – with former world champion Alex Arthur – and punching those pads really is an incredible way to release the aggression. I'd recommend it to anyone who needs an outlet for their pent-up energies.

Experts talk about 'calming', 'expression' and 'suppression' as approaches we can all use to deal with anger. Calming refers to the way in which you can give the emotion time to recede. This could include counting to 10, taking a time out, walking right away or even just inhaling deeply.

These tactics can create room for either expression, where you explain the issue in a clear and assertive but respectful manner (this is usually viewed as the most effective course of action), or suppression, which doesn't mean holding it in, because that can have its own negative consequences, but dealing with it internally without getting agitated. Understanding others' motivations, finding a positive aspect of an argument to focus on or even putting it down to experience can all help if they truly dissolve the anger.

32. Losing control

It might seem a sure-fire route to anxiety central, but allowing yourself to lose control – accepting surprises, appreciating imperfection and going with the flow – should be liberating.

Control freak. It doesn't have many positive associations, does it? OK, people can bully and manipulate to get things done the way they want and that's not good, but for many it's actually just a desire for a certain amount of order in life. Yep – you guessed – I'm what some might call a control freak. On the face of it, that's a good thing. I like to be organised, have a routine and do things correctly, and all those certainly help in both training and in running a business.

There's only one problem with it – other people. They might have their own routines, their own ideas of how to do things and their own plans, and there's a fair chance they won't fit in with mine. That can cause tension. Here's an example. I call a girlfriend sometime in the week. 'What are we going to do this weekend?' I ask. 'Oh, I don't know,' she replies. 'Let's just see what happens'. Now that's not good for me. I want to know what and when. If I didn't taken steps to keep the freak in line, I'd be heading for trouble.

Is perfection possible?

Staying in control is hard work; it can be exhausting and stressful. You constantly strive for perfection and are disappointed when you, or others, don't come up to scratch. You don't like to delegate or let others help, so you end up overworking, and you also have a tendency to try to exert control over other's lives. But there is another way: it's called compromise.

Compromise can be a difficult concept to embrace for anyone who likes to order their life. It means letting go and allowing things to be done differently. It means accepting that it's not all about you, unscheduled events may happen, people may let you down and everything might turn to chaos. If you're something of a control freak, I'm not saying this is easy, but if you're more chilled and forget about your fear of the unknown, I think your relationships with other people will improve. We're all different and it would be boring if we weren't.

Just play it cool

'What time you coming over, babe?' 'About 7pm,' she replies. Now, I know that means anytime from 7 to 8.30pm. I've got two choices. I can expect her at 7, then pace up and down for an hour or so, checking the time every five minutes and bawl her out when she finally arrives. Or I can relax and get on with something, knowing she'll arrive sooner or later – it doesn't really matter. Hopefully she'll realise that there will be times when she needs to be prompt and will make an effort. That's compromise.

Ways to let it go

▶ Embrace uncertainty. Surprises can be fun and exciting.

▶ Understand that there is more than one way to do most things.

▶ Accept that you can't control everything. It can be so liberating.

▶ If you're not in control, it doesn't necessarily mean the worst is going to happen.

▶ Keep the ego in check. You might not be as great as you think you are.

33. Avoid burnout

Total burnout is stress's big knockout punch. Don't walk into it. Spot the signs and take some urgent action.

If one thing defines me, it's that I'm a hard worker. I don't like to stop while there are still things to do – and there are always things to do! There are times when I've worked seven days a week and 16 hours a day. My mind couldn't settle and I'd find myself getting out of bed and going to the office at 3 or 4am.

For someone working to improve people's health, I wasn't being a great role model and, although deep down I knew it wasn't right, I couldn't see an alternative. Finally, there came a point where things started to go wrong. I was becoming unproductive and I found it harder and harder to motivate myself. I was approaching burnout.

Burnout is a thing. It's the result of continual pressure and, although mostly associated with work, it can be related to any stressful activity. Mental and physical exhaustion are obvious symptoms, but burnout is especially characterised by demotivation and cynicism. These can spread from a feeling of dissatisfaction with your job to a detachment from your loved ones or friends. Quite simply, nothing – and no one – seems worth the effort.

Solutions do exist

I was my own boss. For me the answer was relatively straightforward, if not easy. I gave myself a break. I stopped working stupidly long hours, I made time to switch off at the end of the day and had at least one day a week completely away from work. As a result, I was able to manage my time better and become more productive, and quite quickly I began to feel like I was back in charge of my own life again.

If you're working in an intense environment or have a crazy, demanding job, it's going to be more difficult to extract yourself from potential burnout. It is, however, super-important that you make every effort you possibly can. Apart from protecting your own physical and mental health, an exhausted, disaffected worker is no use to any company.

Strategies to stop the collapse

▶ **Talk to managers or HR** about your situation and try to solve workload issues.

▶ **Take two or three 10 to 15-minute breaks in the day.** Use them to relax; sit quietly, go for a stroll or read (but preferably not on your phone).

▶ **Switch off from work when you finish.** Do something completely different and avoid screens if you spend long hours during the day working at a computer.

▶ **Exercise.** You may not feel like it, but force yourself, even if it's a brisk walk or a short 10-minute workout. Focus solely on your body and how your body feels rather than any stressful thoughts.

▶ **Eat regularly and healthily.** Make time for proper balanced meals with plenty of vegetables and protein.

▶ **Allocate 'me time'.** At least once a day, make sure you do just what you want to do, whether that's calling a friend, watching TV or baking a cake.

▶ **Sleep like a baby**. Have a fixed bedtime, wind down a bit beforehand and get a minimum of seven or eight hours' sleep in.

WELCOME TO *LOVE ISLAND*

By February 2019 I had split with my girlfriend of over a year and, when I changed my Facebook status to 'single', it didn't take long for the *Love Island* production company to get back in touch. They had kept on eye on me and wanted to know if I was now ready to audition. It was time to weigh up the pros and cons. The series had been a launch pad to celebrity status for former islanders such as Alex and Olivia Bowen, Dani Dyer, Kem Cetinay and Chris Brown. They now made a good living as social media influencers, models and TV presenters, as well as through their fashion and cosmetic product endorsements. However, I now had a thriving business of my own, which I loved. I didn't need the money and didn't have the time or the inclination to be a full-time celebrity.

My original motivation was to go on TV to raise my profile in order to promote my kids' fitness DVD. The DVD era had now come to a close, but transforming the original plan to suit an app opened up more opportunities. It was a different technology, but there was more I could do with it – and a spell in the limelight would still help it reach more children. As for finding love, I was enjoying being on my own for the first extended period since I was 15. I certainly wasn't looking to find a new girlfriend on the show, but I was single now and if I had a little fun it wouldn't hurt anyone.

Although the producers had called me, I still had to go through the same audition process as everyone else, starting with a one-minute video about myself. I had no idea what they were looking for and searched in vain for previous islanders' videos, so I just went for it. I shot it in the kitchen at the Ranch, just wearing some jeans and a plain blue top, and became cocky Anton, the boy with the banter.

Comparing relationships to chocolate bars, I explained that Galaxy might be your favourite, but you don't want it all the time. You might fancy a Dairy Milk or even two at the same time with a Twix. I went on to say the villa would be my chocolate factory, I'd be Willy Wonka and if I didn't win the golden ticket I'd definitely have some fun with the Oompa Loompas!

I sent it off, but didn't forget about it. Before I even heard back, I put in my phone calendar for 3 June: 'First day of *Love Island*'. This was February, four months earlier, when they still had 150,000 applications to sift. I visualised myself on the show, felt certain I would be there and willed myself to be selected.

> **WHEN I WATCH THE VIDEO BACK NOW, PART OF ME CRINGES, BUT I'M ALSO KIND OF PROUD, BECAUSE I NAILED IT. I WAS EXACTLY WHAT THEY WANTED. IT PORTRAYED ME AS A CONFIDENT CHARACTER WITH A SENSE OF HUMOUR AND AN EYE FOR THE GIRLS.**

When I watch the video back now, part of me cringes, but I'm also kind of proud, because I nailed it. I was exactly what they wanted. It portrayed me as a confident character with a sense of humour and an eye for the girls. The producers later said it was the best audition video they had ever seen. Sure enough, I got the call to go to Manchester to meet the casting directors – I was now down to the last 1000. When I went into the waiting room, I took my place among the other applicants. I looked along the line, and to a boy they were all showing off their muscles in their skin-tight shirts. I'd worn a suit jacket. They had seen the photos of me, they knew what I looked like and I was pleased to be presenting something different. I went in last and, pointing back at them, told the producers, 'Someone's been shopping in the kids' section!'

They talked about my exes, my dating history and my life in general. They were used to the pretty Essex boy type, and I had something different to offer. They hadn't had a Scottish lad on the show before and few who were already running their own successful business. At the end I had to look down the camera and say something about myself for the executive producers who had the final say. Why waste a good idea, I thought, so I repeated the Willy Wonka line. Some of the production team hadn't seen my original video and I could hear them laughing as I spoke. That made me feel like I was walking on air. A little later my friend rang to see how it went. I had no doubt and let him know in just three words: 'I smashed it!'

Two weeks later, I was meeting the exec producers. They were now paying me expenses and they sent a guy to meet me at the station holding a card with an ITV logo and my name on it – I was getting close. I knew if I got this far, I could talk my way on to the show. I gave an exaggerated version of the real me. I was Ants with the bants, the Scottish lad, a real charmer with a relaxed, open attitude to relationships. How could they resist?

I got the call I had been waiting for. They liked me and I'd been picked – as a 'bombshell'. That wasn't in my script. Bombshells are contestants dropped in unexpectedly during the show to add drama and disrupt the cosy couples in the villa. They don't enter the villa on 3 June, the date I'd put in my diary months earlier. I had even scheduled my 12-week diet based on that very date. I should have been ecstatic about being selected. My mum tried to put the positive side, pointing out that as a bombshell all the focus is on you. Rather than sharing the stage with 30 others, you get the spotlight. But I still couldn't hide my disappointment.

A couple of weeks before the show begins, the contestants are brought to London for a media day to record promotional videos and photoshoots. I knew enough about the show to know that only starters took part, not bombshells. I was there, so was I a starter now? No one could tell me. The security was now fully operational. I had a chaperone with a walkie-talkie, who radioed ahead to make sure I didn't see any of the other contestants as I headed to the room to record my intro video.

There were cameras everywhere and 50 or more people watching as they stood me in front of a wall of my Instagram pics. For the first time since the process began, the nerves really kicked in. My voice was shaking and I just couldn't focus on what I was saying. I was making mistakes and the jokes I tried to make didn't come out right – I just sounded arrogant. I kept apologising, but the producers were having none of it. 'Don't worry. They'll love you,' they said. 'Do you know who did the worst-ever intro video? Kem!' And he went on to win *Love Island*. Still, I felt deflated. If they choose who starts on that performance, I had no chance.

I had the medical – a pretty in-depth check-up with STD and blood tests – and saw the psychiatrist, who told me I came across as a well-put-together young man. A week later I got the call. In four days' time I would be picked up and taken to the airport to get on a flight to Majorca. It was really happening. I was bursting to tell the whole world, but I was warned that if the news leaked out I wouldn't be on the show. So I told just my mum and dad, knowing they could keep a secret.

> IT WAS REALLY HAPPENING. I WAS BURSTING TO TELL THE WHOLE WORLD, BUT I WAS WARNED THAT IF THE NEWS LEAKED OUT I WOULDN'T BE ON THE SHOW. SO I TOLD JUST MY MUM AND DAD, KNOWING THEY COULD KEEP A SECRET.

As soon as I landed in Majorca, they took my phone from me. From now on I was in lockdown with no more communication with the outside world. There I was, thinking that as a bombshell I could be facing three weeks of this when my chaperone received a text from the producers. It said that I was to be a starter after all. I was buzzing. Just as I began to have doubts, my dream had come true.

The week went by in a blur. It was a nice hotel apart from their gym, which was terrible. I begged the producers to find me a proper gym and offered to pay for it from the weekly allowance they gave me, and they were kind enough to find one for me. At various times the producers came to check I was OK and to run through the rules. A choice of clothes arrived from the show's favoured brands. You could pick what you wanted, except for the arrival outfit, which a fashion advisor helped select.

I WALKED THROUGH THE DOOR, MET CAROLINE FLACK AND THEN STOOD THERE AS FIVE GIRLS LOOKED ME UP AND DOWN. I STARTED GETTING THE SHAKES, BUT I WAS HERE. I'D MADE IT TO THE VILLA.

I was also lucky with my chaperone, Sam, who stayed with me all week. He helped me feel comfortable and chilled, and made the stay much more fun. I promised I'd get back in touch with him when I got out and I kept my word. His job was to keep me away from any cameras or prying eyes. It wasn't always easy. One day I had to go down to reception to pick up my *Love Island* suitcase. I was taking it back to my bedroom when a group of teenage girls recognised the case and guessed I was a contestant. Sam freaked out and pushed me into the room. They hung around outside the room and, though I felt bad, I had to stay hidden from them. After the show was over, one of them messaged me and I was pleased to be able send them a video message to make amends.

As the day approached, my excitement built. On the actual day the show started I was due to be picked up at 6.30am, but had so much nervous energy I went for a run first. They took me to a different hotel where I was to get ready. The make-up team prepare you so you look OK on camera under the lights, the security team check your case to make sure you're not smuggling anything in, and you're left in the room to wait to be called.

I spent some time visualising the walk-through and then, to calm my nerves, I decided to do few press-ups. I hadn't realised there was some kind of ash on the floor and when I stood up there were brown marks on my shorts. The idea of walking into the villa looking like that was like a nightmare. There was a mad panic as the team scampered around looking for a spare pair. So if you wondered why I chose to enter the villa wearing quite such tight shorts, there's your answer.

Suddenly, the moment arrived. I had reached a state of calm, but discovering I was to be the first boy to enter the villa shook me up again a bit. I walked through the door, met Caroline Flack and then stood there as five girls looked me up and down. I started getting the shakes, but I was here. I'd made it to the villa.

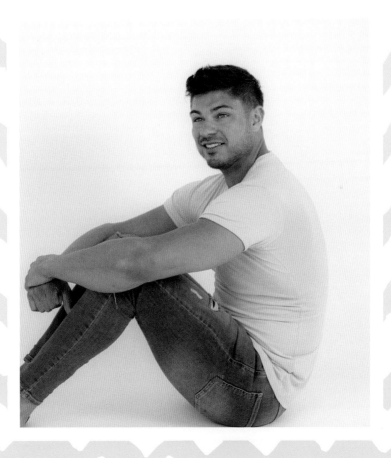

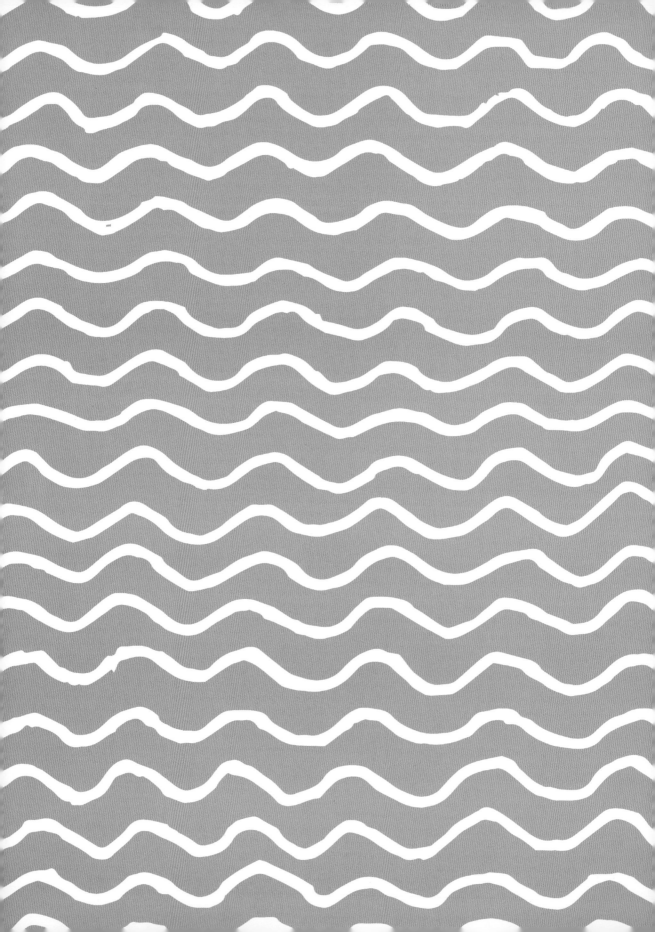

Be happy

Smile at the world, and it will smile back. You will be amazed at how much a positive attitude, a belief in yourself and an acceptance of life's setbacks can boost your own ambitions and your sense of contentment.

34. Happiness is allowed

It's true that it's easier for some people than others, and of course we all have difficult days and down times, but you don't need anyone else's permission. It's up to you. Happiness is something you can actively choose.

I'm naturally a cheerful guy. When I was on *Love Island*, I'd start the day by announcing 'Another day in paradise!' – and I meant it. I wake up excited about what's to come and I face most of the challenges, chores and surprises in life with the same enthusiasm. It's true that I've got plenty to be pleased about right now – a loving family, a job I enjoy, a secure income – but, like everyone, I've also had worries, disappointments and difficulties to cope with.

Finding that inner contentment isn't always easy. Modern life puts so many pressures and expectations on us, it feels natural to be weighed down by it all. It isn't, though – that's just the stuff surrounding life, it isn't life itself. If you let these things get to you, they will, but if you can see beyond them to enjoy being you and the good things you have going, you can get so much more out of life. It starts by allowing yourself to be happy. It's a strong and attractive characteristic, and I like myself for having it, but I've also found other people like me for it too.

Embrace it all

Life is going to throw all kinds of everything at you. Sadness and grief are part of that, but they will pass and they don't need to define who you are. Take it all in, the good and the bad, as part of an incredible life-long rollercoaster ride.

If you want to change your appearance, your lifestyle or your attitude, go ahead. I'm all for self-criticism, but don't let it be your guiding

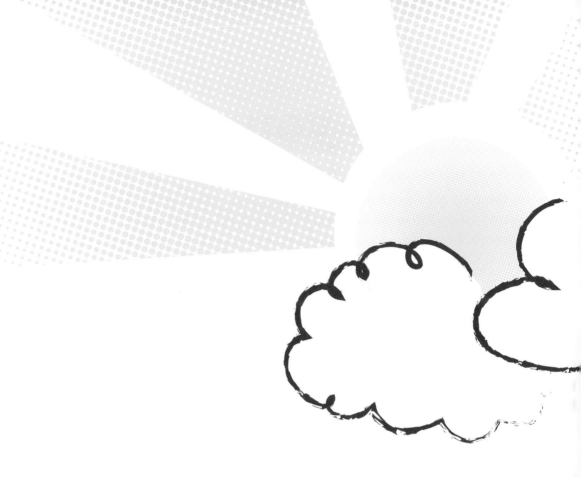

characteristic. Allow yourself to make mistakes, to have bad habits or fail. Admit you (like everyone else) are not perfect and get over it. Talk to yourself as if you were a friend, with understanding, compassion and encouragement.

Value what you have

Try listing the things you do have, especially those things you can't touch like love, friendship and health. They're worth so much more than all the things you don't. Of course, there's bound to be lots of things that you really, really want, but what you already have should be more than enough to make you happy.

I think it's really important to keep a sense of proportion. There's always going to be something that will bother you, if you let it. But you really don't have to. Arguments, disappointments, things you've lost and things you didn't want to happen – sooner or later they will all be washed away by the events of life, so mentally process them and then move on.

35. Be your best self

We can all realise our potential, feel good about ourselves, maximise our happiness and live a fulfilling life. We might need to be bold, work hard and sometimes accept failure, but if we don't move our lives forward, then who will?

'Just be yourself.' They say that in films, don't they, when a character feels misunderstood or left out. If you stop trying to be cool, or one of the gang, and accept the way you are, things will turn out OK. Except it doesn't really work like that. However, I do think you can try to be the best possible version of you. That's a you who sets goals and strives to reach them, has a moral code and sticks by it, and is not afraid of new challenges. Instead of accepting who you are, I believe you should take responsibility for who you are, what you do and where you want to be.

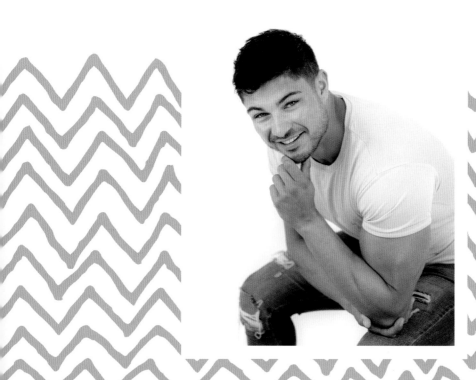

Nothing will happen if you stand and wait, though. The sooner you realise that only you can make your wishes, ambitions, even your wildest dreams, come true, the better. Only then can you begin to work out what you need to do to get there. Don't accept defeat and never stop planning. If you hit a dead end, turn around and discover another route. If one dream doesn't come true, then start on another. There's no limit on the number of dreams you're allowed.

Be someone else

But you don't have to accept the way you are. There are so many things about your character that you can change and still be 'you'. You might try to become friendlier, kinder, fitter, more hard-working, more respectful or less argumentative – and that might lead you to find a self that you are happier being.

Part of that is never being afraid to try something new or different. There could be an aspect of your personality that you haven't encountered yet, but the only way you're going to find out is by stepping out of your comfort zone and challenging yourself. It might be asking out that person you think is out of your league, requesting more responsibility from your boss or putting yourself on display – perhaps performing or speaking in public.

Healthy approach

Feeling good about yourself starts with your mind and body. Give yourself time to think about yourself and what's going on in your life. Savour those things that make you happy and try to understand why you might be worried or sad, and what you can do about it. Physical health is just as important. Regular exercise has the power to boost self-esteem, reduce anxiety and increase our levels of energy and positivity.

What is it that's distracting you in life? It could be a bad relationship, overcritical parents, your own lack of confidence or even an instinct to put others first. It won't just disappear, so find a way to block out the negative noise and make you own path.

Be proud of every single achievement, no matter how small. As nice as it is to receive congratulations from others, learn to appreciate your own judgement about your accomplishments. These are the steps to building self-confidence and they'll give you the strength to progress in your life goals.

36. It happens for a reason

It's not that I necessarily believe there's a divine plan, a guiding force directing my life, but I do believe that the events of our lives, both good and bad, happen so that we can benefit from them.

My attitude to life was brilliantly summed up by the actor Jim Carrey when he spoke about making sense of the apparent chaos of life. 'When I say life doesn't happen to you, it happens for you, I really don't know if that's true,' he said. 'I'm just making a conscious choice to perceive challenges as something beneficial so that I can deal with them in the most productive way.'

Finding meaning

Personally, I don't believe in destiny or fate, because for me believing that everything happens for a reason is about finding meaning in, and learning from, both our positive and negative experiences. If something went well, how did you contribute to the success? How can you replicate those actions in future? How does it make you feel about your own abilities?

After a bad event, perhaps an argument, a relationship breakdown or an unsuccessful job interview, be honest with yourself about your own failings. If you were able to rewind time, what would you do differently? What can you do to make sure you act better in future?

Opening up to disappointment

Long before I was asked to apply for *Love Island*, I auditioned for a similar, if less popular show, *Survival of the Fittest*, but I did hardly any preparation. I really wasn't clued up as to what the series was about and what kind of person they might be looking for, so when it came to the interview I completely froze and, when I did manage to speak, I was nervous and didn't make a lot of sense.

Naturally, they turned me down. I was disappointed, but it wasn't a waste of time. There were so many lessons I took from that experience, including the need for preparation, how I would project my personality and what impression I wanted to leave. When the time to audition for *Love Island* came around, I used all this to my advantage.

It's your response that matters

Remember that we are only able to control our responses to other people's behaviour. The person interviewing me may not have been friendly or engaging enough, but blaming them wasn't an option, because I had no control over what they did. I could only ask myself how I could have reacted differently.

Guilt is the other side of that coin. If we regret our actions we can apologise or try to make amends, but carrying that guilt without understanding what we learned about ourselves is only going to hamper our progression.

Creating meaning from your experiences is not just rewarding, but incredibly satisfying. When you reach a crossroads, a crisis or an opportunity and realise that your life has prepared you for that very moment, it can make you feel so confident and strong that you will understand why some people do call it destiny.

37. Dream on...

Visualisation is like a dream where you're in control of what happens. Using your own imagination you can create a scene or a series of events which can help you relax, achieve and change your emotions.

Our minds are constantly running through alternative scenarios. *What if I miss the train? What will that kiss feel like? What shall I have for dinner?* As they do that, they throw up various images, which help us process our thoughts. It happens so often we don't even notice, but we can use that same power to focus our mind.

Like everything a little practice helps. Give yourself a few quiet minutes now and then to hone your visualisation skills. Begin with something you're familiar with, like your journey to work or cooking your favourite meal. Take it slowly, making sure you have a clear picture of each step with as many details as possible. Details are the key, as it's the little things that make the scenario believable. Be sure to include emotions in your visualisation – are you happy, scared, excited? – to make them as realistic as you can.

Once you feel you've mastered the ability to create and hold a picture in your mind, try imagining something familiar, but which hasn't happened yet – perhaps you scoring a goal or making friends laugh. When you're able to immerse yourself in a visualisation and hold your concentration, you will begin to trick your subconscious into thinking that these scenes are real. That opens up a number of opportunities for you to control and change your mindset.

Three areas where visualisation is helpful

Mood: This is the 'happy place' scenario. Think of a scene you can repeatedly conjure up of a time or place – real or imagined – when you felt contented and relaxed. The obvious example is a beach paradise, but it could be a party, a walk in the woods or watching a favourite film. The key is what emotions that scene evokes in you. The more you bring the picture forward, the more your brain will automatically generate those feelings of happiness and serenity when you feel most anxious or stressed.

Confidence: The ability to clearly imagine yourself in a situation where you have proved yourself, achieved a goal or overcome fears and obstacles is invaluable in summoning confidence and strength. Again, it should be a clear picture that you have repeatedly imagined and immediately associate with success. Next time you're nervous or scared, use this visualisation as part of your preparation.

Goals: Fulfilling an objective makes use of that ability to create detailed, imagined pictures of future events. The more you feel your visualisation is a reality, the greater the boost it will provide. You can use it to plot a series of steps on the way to your eventual goal, and it can help enable you to rehearse how you'll act in certain situations along that journey. Work hard to create that vision of you achieving your final goal. Knowing how success feels and how much it means to you will be a fantastic source of motivation.

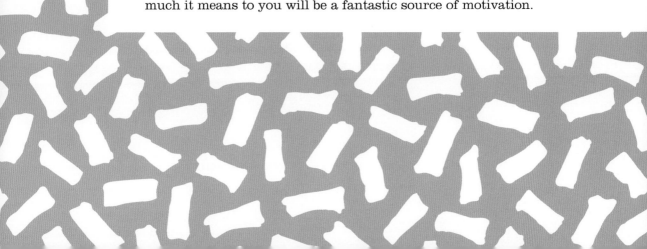

38. Attract happiness

If you believe in something enough, you can make it happen. According to the law of attraction, good thoughts bring good fortune and unleash the mind's great potential to bring about change.

As soon as I sent my audition video in to the *Love Island* production company I went straight to my phone and made a diary entry. For 3 June I wrote, 'First day of *Love Island*'. It was February, four months before that date. Never mind the 150,000 other applicants and the whole set of hurdles I would have to clear before being selected for the show, in my mind I was certain I would be stepping into the villa on the first day of the show.

There's this theory called the law of attraction, which says that positive thoughts lead to positive outcomes and negative thoughts bring about negative consequences – or, in other words, that happiness causes happy things to happen. It's basically about believing in self-fulfilment – if you focus your thoughts on anything, you can turn them into reality. The idea is that it utilises the power of the mind to produce an energy that can attract the thing we wish for into our mind. It might be a new relationship, a new job or a new car.

Ask, believe, receive

Rhonda Byrne's book *The Secret*, which builds on this notion to explain how positivity, visualisation and willpower can be used as a means of making dreams a reality, made a real impression on me. *The Secret* describes a three-step process: ask, believe and receive. That is to say, understand precisely what you want, set about achieving your goal with the certainty that you will succeed and be open to the paths

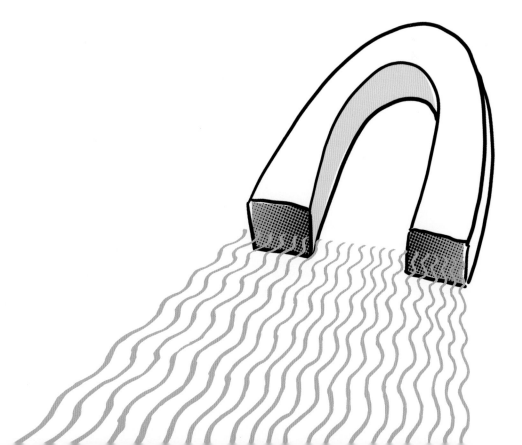

which will help you. The asking and receiving parts can be easy; the believing is often difficult. It requires complete positivity (part of the deal is that negative thoughts attract negative outcomes) and an ability to be continually convinced of your eventual success, despite any setbacks or diversions.

It might not tally with the science you learned at school and not everyone buys into this process, but plenty of people cite examples where it has resulted in success. Whatever your view, though, there is little doubting the power of the mind to shape your emotions and your circumstances. I certainly believe that concentrating on what you want or where you want to be, with the confidence that it will definitely happen, can only enhance your feelings of motivation, determination and focus, both consciously and subconsciously, so I'd say why not give it a try?

THE *LOVE ISLAND* EXPERIENCE

In the spring of 2019, as the *Love Island* interview process ran its course, I worked hard on my preparation. I was going to look as good as I ever had and underwent a 12-week diet that would really show off my six-pack. I also worked my way through all four of the previous seasons of the show and analysed who I liked and why, the potential pitfalls and the opportunities to make a good impression.

So I went into the villa confident that if I didn't win the show I could still be a popular contestant. Luckily, I didn't know what was happening back home. My intro video had not gone down well. Lines like, 'It's not my body or my looks that gets the women into bed – it's my banter' had not sounded funny, which is what I had intended. I came across as arrogant and that 'severe medical condition' called 'a wandering eye' made me sound as if I was a love cheat. While I was feeling my way into the show, the tabloids were busy digging up all kinds of dirt on me. I was branded 'an embarrassment to Scotland' and there was even a petition to bring me home. I was the bookies' favourite to be the first person eliminated at odds of 4/5 – virtually a certainty!

I might not have realised how bad it was looking for me at home, but in the villa things were not going brilliantly either. I was determined to make the most of my time out there. Whereas some of the contestants were sometimes reticent and scared of making fools of themselves, I threw myself into it. On the first day, when we finally got to bed at 4am, I looked around and exclaimed, 'Boys, this is going to be great!' And it was.

There's always a lot of talk about which of the islanders are 'playing a game' and who is for real. I can't really speak about others' intentions, but this was my attitude: I wanted to do well on the show and had an idea of what I had to do to win it. Mostly though, I really wanted to have a full-on *Love Island* experience, whether that meant drama, laughs, romance or just adventures that would never be repeated. I kept that mentality while I was there, but the intensity of the experience is phenomenal. When you're living that closely and under such scrutiny, emotions become heightened and you can almost forget you are even in a reality show.

I CAME ACROSS AS ARROGANT AND THE 'SEVERE MEDICAL CONDITION' CALLED 'A WANDERING EYE' MADE ME SOUND AS IF I WAS A LOVE CHEAT.

I had a great time in that first week. I palled up with Joe and Michael as they came in early too, but I can honestly say I got on with everyone on the show. I was disappointed when Joe left in the second week because he was my go-to guy in the villa, but that was part of the game. Unfortunately for me, so was the coupling. I knew almost immediately that Amy, who I had chosen when I entered the villa, was not for me and decided to try my chances with Lucie. That didn't play out well. It ended with me being pied and, as I discovered when I got home, being vilified on social media. I was a snake and a love rat, but all I'd done was slightly upset someone I'd only known for a few hours!

No one wants to be the first to leave the island, and my chances of staying beyond five days looked slim. The first eviction came after a re-coupling in which each girl would choose a boy to pair up with: the one who remained single would be dumped and sent packing. My only hope came from Anna, who I had bonded with in those early days. She could tell I was fearing the worst and, with a knowing smile, told me not to worry. When it came to her turn to choose she started talking about who she was going to pick. Joe whispered to me, 'I think it's you!' and when she started talking about his sexy body even I was convinced. When she called out Sherif, my face dropped a mile. That was it. I was going home.

It turned out I was being royally pranked. The girls had cooked up a plan for Amber to save me because they liked having me around. Amber wasn't romantically interested in me – she even built a wall of pillows between us when we shared a bed. I think she saw me more as an annoying little brother, but thanks to her I remained in the villa. It was a massive relief and I vowed to relax and just enjoy the journey from here on in.

In that first week I had shared a conversation with Yewande, who was feeling insecure about not being among the boys' first picks. I told her how I was used to being 'first pick' back home, but had to get used to being pied on the show. 'I know that just because I'm not someone's initial type doesn't mean that I'm a bad-looking guy or a bad guy or anything', I explained. And then I told her, 'And you just need to feel the same.' She was lovely and just needed a boost of confidence. I even gave her my *Wolf of Wall Street* chest-beating!

This was the real me and gradually more of that was emerging. I felt more comfortable and was winning viewers around too. When Elma joined the show, she picked me to cook her main meal at the dinner date. I cooked up a wicked carbonara and we were soon coupled up. I really think we could have stayed together – she's still a good friend now – but the next vote saw us picked as one of the two most incompatible couples. The public voted for two from those couples to be dumped and they chose Elma and Joe. I'd always wondered why islanders cry at these moments, when they will see these people again in a matter of weeks, but I blubbed then – I'd lost my best mate and a girl I was getting on really well with.

In the next re-coupling, I picked Lucie. It was just because we already had a friendship, but nevertheless I realised that back home Joe would be angry with both of us. He later told me that he was indeed fuming, but calmed down once he saw that Lucie just wanted to stay on the show. So did I, but the show was about coupling up. I was still loving everything about the villa – the challenges, the food, the banter – but after three weeks I'd been pied, overlooked for other guys and I still hadn't kissed a girl! So it was completely astounding when Lucie and I survived the public vote as one of the three most popular couples. I still get goosebumps thinking about that moment when I realised that I had been accepted by the viewers.

THIS WAS THE REAL ME AND GRADUALLY MORE OF THAT WAS EMERGING. I FELT MORE COMFORTABLE AND WAS WINNING VIEWERS AROUND TOO.

The very next day – buoyed by the vote – they introduced five new girls at Casa Amor. 'Five,' I told myself. 'Even you can't mess this up!' Fortunately, I met Belle and we clicked. Things got even better when Craig David appeared to give a Ministry of Sound show. I've been a massive fan of his for years and been out to Ibiza to see him. Those tears of happiness I shed on seeing him there were real. And it led to the only time I broke the Island rules. I'd been called to the beach hut to talk about my reactions to his show, but as I made my way there I came across Craig and the producers. Now, we were under strict instructions not to touch anyone, so when I saw him hold his fist out to me, I glanced at the producers. They shook their heads to say, 'Don't you dare,' but I was buzzing so I ignored them, jumped across and fist-bumped him. On Day 36, Belle and I went on our first date. I might have broken the show's record for not finding a partner, but once I did, I felt like nothing could stop me.

The producers liked me because I was always aware that the show was about entertainment and tried to make things interesting. When they picked the biggest jokers – Tommy, Jordan and I – for a trip to the shops, I tried to live up to the tag. Just for a laugh, I pretended to give the cashier my number. As far as the viewers were concerned, Anton the snake was back, even though when Belle found out she really wasn't that bothered (she knew I had no phone in the villa and had just made up a number), but was encouraged to show she was annoyed.

I wasn't so lucky on the second occasion. We were playing a game of 'snog, marry, pie'. The girls went first and all chose to kiss the person they were coupled up with, and marry and pie the obvious candidates. The producers thought it was so boring and took the boys aside, telling us to liven things up. I was first up and Belle knew I'd do what I was told. 'Don't you f***ing dare,' she mouthed to me. I went ahead and kissed Anna – it was only a bit of fun. The show might want fun, but it needs drama too. Belle was riled, hyped up by the producers, and we were told we had to have a conversation about it. Belle ripping into me was great TV, but I felt humiliated and the most embarrassed I'd ever been. I was raging, but remembering that similar situation on *Glow*, kept telling myself: 'Don't react, just don't react.'

> **BELLE RIPPING INTO ME WAS GREAT TV, BUT I FELT HUMILIATED AND THE MOST EMBARRASSED I'D EVER BEEN. I WAS RAGING, BUT KEPT TELLING MYSELF: 'DON'T REACT, JUST DON'T REACT.'**

No sooner had we made up than I found myself in hospital. I had a slight fever and a stomach pain and was rushed off by the *Love Island* team. It was so weird being in a hospital bed with my family not even knowing and a security guard sitting by my side! They feared I had appendicitis, but it was just dehydration from working out in the heat and drinking too much coffee and after two days on a drip I was back for the final week.

The last 10 days were great. Belle and I were getting on really well; the challenges, especially looking after the pretend baby, were fun; and we had a thrilling final date in which we took a helicopter ride over the island and enjoyed a picnic in a stunning cove. Who wouldn't fall a little in love in such an intense situation and such beautiful surroundings? It could only be capped by winning the series.

Leaving on a public vote on the penultimate day was so gutting. I really believed we had a chance of winning. Later, when the disappointment wore off, I realised I was a winner. I had gone for the *Love Island* experience and had a 100% blast. I was the first boy to enter and one of the last to leave, and I enjoyed a whirlwind 56-day rollercoaster of emotions, challenges, laughter and tears. I will never forget *Love Island 2019*.

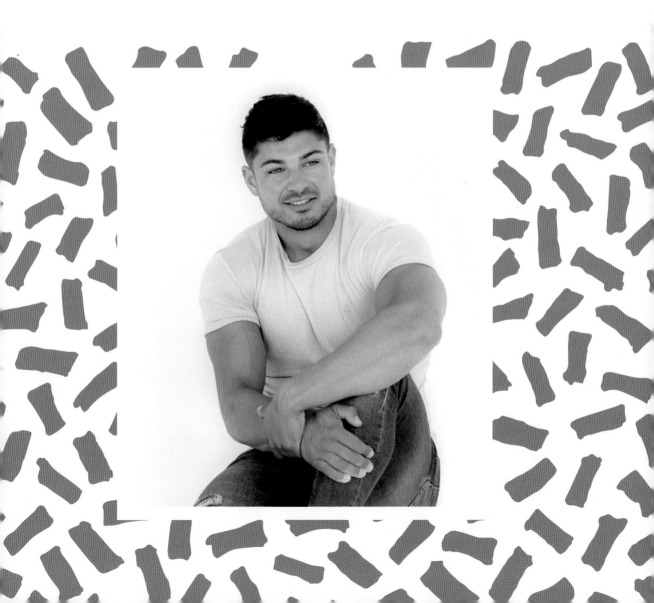

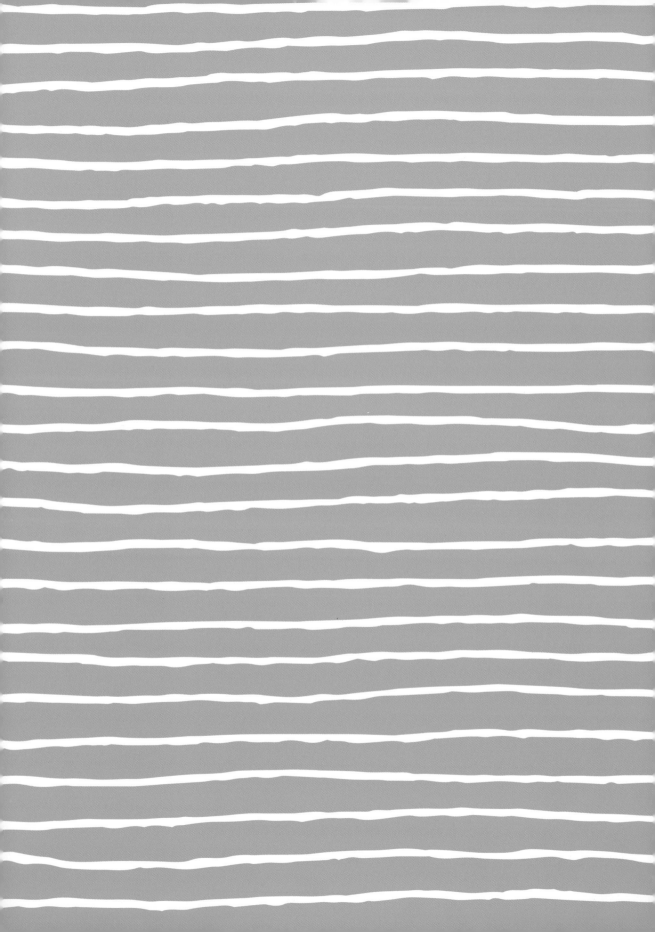

Lifestyle

Health and happiness begins with you. From personal grooming to social media and sleep, choosing to live your life with self-respect, a sense of calm and a certain amount of order will benefit your body and your mind.

39. Taking care of yourself

Personal hygiene is the bedrock of self-esteem. Adopting a self-care routine not only ensures you stay clean and healthy, but allows you to flourish and thrive.

You have to look after yourself. You are all you've got. That begins with personal hygiene, but how we feel physically is related to our mental health. Building essential self-care routines into our day is a statement of self-worth. It's amazing how the simple actions of caring for our bodies can improve our mood and motivation.

Look, I'm sure you don't really need me to tell you how to do this stuff, but just in case there are any areas you're forgetting, here's a run-down of my approach to keeping myself healthy not just on the outside, but on the inside too, because they're so closely linked.

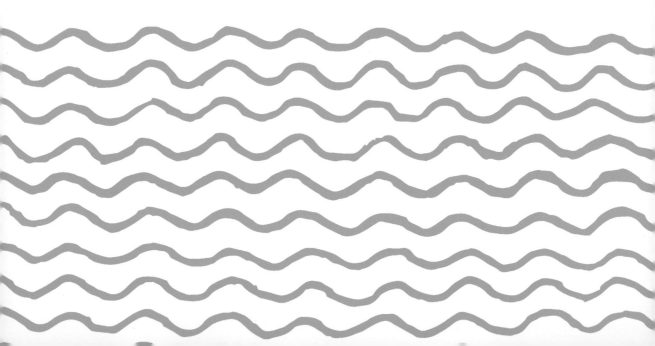

Head to toe hygiene

Shower: It all starts with cleanliness. Shower every morning and again later after you exercise or if you're heading out with company.

Hands: If the Covid-19 pandemic has taught us nothing else, it has hammered home how important it is to wash your hands regularly and effectively. Washing your hands after you visit the toilet and before you eat are essentials, but we should also be aware that we touch our faces over 15 times an hour. Use hand sanitiser when you're out and wash as soon as you come inside.

Teeth: Brushing your teeth twice a day should be part of your daily routine. As well as keeping your teeth healthy, that feeling of fresh breath is deep-seated and is a potent signal to our brains that we're feeling bright and clean.

Nails: If other people don't look at our hands, we do. They are the parts of you that you can see without a mirror and can be a constant reminder of how you feel. A manicure can give you a great boost, but it costs nothing to keep them clean and tidy yourself.

Hair: Just the fact that we talk about 'bad hair days' shows how important hair is to our self-esteem. Regular washing, combing and trims to avoid split ends will keep your hair in good condition, but it's also worth considering how different styles make you feel about yourself.

Skin: Don't rely on make-up to hide skin problems. Establish a daily skincare routine that leaves your skin in the best possible condition. And remember, drinking plenty of water and eating a healthy diet will do more for your skin than all the cream in the world.

Go outside: Being out in the open air has many benefits for mental health, but, importantly, sunlight is the major source of vitamin D, which is key to helping teeth, muscles and bones healthy.

Exercise: I can't repeat it enough: regular exercise is essential for your short- and long-term physical health. You don't have to kill yourself working out every day if you don't want to, though. Just do 30 minutes of moderate exercise four times a week.

Diet: Our daily food choices are key to our physical health and wellbeing. Only a balanced diet can supply the nutrients and hydration our bodies need to survive, and our energy levels, moods and continued health rely on eating sensibly.

40. Make it routine

Having a structure to your day is another of the secrets to success. In my view it's the route to achieving and satisfaction – and, no, routine doesn't mean boring. Honestly.

I simply can't stress enough how central a sense of routine is to my feeling of wellbeing. It helps me feel that I'm in control, that I'm working towards my goals, and it reduces my stress levels. The lockdowns during the Covid pandemic made life difficult for me, as they did for many people, but I reacted to the disruption they caused by adopting a routine and sticking to it. It really helped me get through and, to be honest, it was a relief to get back to having a rhythm to my day.

My old routines had been wrecked by my time in *Love Island* and the subsequent changes to my lifestyle. I was all over the place in my work patterns, my eating and my sleeping. Days could drift by when the only thing I actually had to do was make sure I arrived for a personal appearance on time. Without any order in my life, it was so easy for boredom and laziness to kick in.

Having a daily routine doesn't mean you're chained to doing the same thing every day or that you can never do anything spontaneous. In fact, one of the greatest bonuses of having a routine is the thrill of breaking it. However, to break it you need to have it in the first place! All I'm talking about is having a set pattern to your day so that you can split up your time to achieve certain goals.

Your own routine will be dictated by work and family commitments, but keeping to the following guidelines can help you build a structure into your day.

Creating a framework

Rise and shine: Set you alarm for the same time every day and make sure you shower and dress immediately. This prepares you mentally and physically for the day ahead. If you want to give yourself an extra hour in bed at the weekends, then do!

Daily schedule: Before you begin the day, consider what needs to be achieved and build a schedule to achieve those goals. If you have a plan, you are less likely to fritter time away or forget about important deadlines.

Mealtimes: Your breakfast, lunch and dinner provide the energy for your activities and help break up the day. They are a time to relax and, if possible, get together with family, friends or colleagues. Eating at regular times ensures you don't skip meals (which can lead to lower energy levels or bingeing) and makes it easier for you to timetable meetings and appointments.

Hydrate: Staying hydrated is essential to avoid fatigue, to keep your joints supple and nourish your skin. You should drink water regularly throughout the day. Around six to eight tumblers should be enough, perhaps more if it's hot or you're exercising. Drink at meal times and when you're thirsty, but if you're forgetful build more set times into your daily schedule.

Exercise: Remember to build time into your routine to exercise. It's as important for your wellbeing as food and sleep, but it's often the casualty of a busy day or a day without focus.

Bedtime: Stick to a consistent time to go to sleep. Your body will respond and you will be more productive the next day. It's all too easy to push the time you set for sleep later and later, which not only leaves you tired, but means one day can drift into another.

41. Looking good

Dressing well won't necessarily guarantee that you succeed in your goals. However, the boost it can give you can certainly help.

I believe in dressing for the occasion. I'll put on a suit and tie for a fancy do, a jacket and smart trousers for a club, T-shirt and jeans if I'm dressing down. Whatever and wherever, though, I never go out looking scruffy. My clothes are cleaned, ironed and smell nice. Since *Love Island* I've been constantly spotted and photographed when I leave the house, so I've been extra careful about my appearance, but I've always liked to dress well. It's a basic. I just wouldn't feel right otherwise.

It's nice when people compliment you on your appearance, what you're wearing or how you smell, but you should look your best for yourself, not for other people. The message it sends out to the world – that you're prepared, that you care and that you value yourself – is also the message you're giving yourself, and it builds your esteem and confidence, and gives you a spring in your step.

Now, I'm not saying you have to look super-fashionable or spend a lot of money. You can invest in expensive designer clothes or purchase an outfit from a high street retailer – either way you can still feel you're presentable and ready to face the world. The important thing is that the clothes fit well, so you feel comfortable, and that they are appropriate for the occasion. Clothes can help you feel relaxed, they can prepare you to focus on work, and they can lift you and put you in the mood for a fun night out.

Smell of success!

Smell plays a massive role in how you're perceived and perceive yourself too. Obviously, it's important to smell fresh and clean. Deodorant after your shower and when you feel hot or flustered can help. Scents can really make a difference to your state of mind. A perfume or cologne can make you feel relaxed, alert, cheerful or even sexy. It's worth experimenting with different fragrances just to see how they make you feel, and you could even build up a selection of scents to suit different moods and occasions. Some people like to have a signature scent that becomes part of their identity. It can be a confident way of announcing yourself and leaving an impression.

Understanding your wardrobe and how it affects how you feel can be a useful way to control your frame of mind. When I am clean-shaven and put on a freshly laundered shirt and a suit, I feel taller. The feeling begins with the ritual of shaving and dressing, and culminates with that check in the mirror. I know it's true of women too, who have their own rituals of putting on a favourite dress, make-up and jewellery. You're dressing for success – and feeling like a winner is the first step to victory.

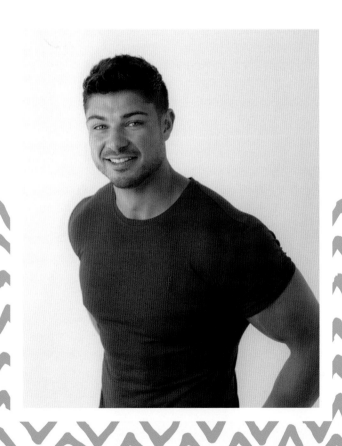

42. Social media

My generation was one of the first to grow up with social media. I love it and it's been important to me professionally, but there can definitely be a downside.

My schooldays coincided with the rise of Bebo, and we loved it. It was fun and never seemed a tool for social pressure, negative comments or bullying – the worst of it was agonising over your Top 16 friends list, who to give your 'luv' to or thinking up something to draw on your whiteboard. Then came Facebook which we filled with holiday pics and chat. By the time I was 17, I was regularly checking my likes and number of friends – I remember limiting my friends to 5000!

At first, I didn't really bother with Instagram, and it was my girlfriend when I was getting the gym underway who encouraged me to post. She was very good-looking and worked in a club, and she had 60,000 followers. I started putting up fitness posts promoting the gym with 12-week transformations, pics and competitions. I went from having 100 followers to getting 3000 likes on a single post and it was brilliant for the business. By the time I left for *Love Island,* I had 4000 followers and I was very happy with that.

On the edge of obsession

When I came out of the villa it had reached 900,000 and soon after that it hit a million. There's money to be made with those kinds of numbers and for a while I tried to adapt my content for the new audience, the ones who came for 'Anton the celebrity' not for fitness advice. I became obsessed with checking my number of followers and it continued to rise. At one point I checked my screen time and it had risen to nine hours a day, so I know how easy it is to get sucked into that world.

I also know how cruel and toxic it can be. I've received so many vicious insults and baseless accusations, especially on Twitter. Sometimes I can just laugh them off, but on other days times I find that harder and they hurt. I'm just amazed by how cruel and nasty people can be.

Reality check

Then it hit me – the people who were abusing me aren't real friends. I took a week off Instagram to try to discover who I was and that led to a six-week absence. When I returned, my posts focused on my fitness and wellbeing message, because that's what I really care about. I reduced my own screen time to nearer two hours and took stock of what I had learned.

Social media and other apps can be brilliant. We can chat, create our own identity, make new friends, find out what's going on and connect with thousands of people, but it's so easy to get drawn in and forget that it's all an illusion and it can even be dangerous to our mental health – so I thought I'd remind you:

▶ **Online life is not real life,** it's a fairy tale world. No one ever posts a bad picture of themselves.

▶ **Don't spend so much time looking at everyone else's life** that you don't consider your own.

▶ **Apps are designed to be addictive.** Cut down your screen time and interact with the real world.

▶ **Social media seems to bring out the cruel side of some people.** Sometimes it's better to switch off the negativity or bullying and walk away.

▶ **Followers and likes are just a finger tap.** Don't mistake them for true friends and real love.

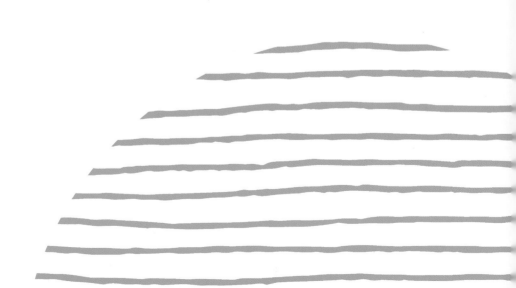

43. Sleep well

A good night's sleep is essential to health and wellbeing. It enables the body to recover from the exertions of the previous day and prepares it for the next one. I love it!

I'm a great sleeper, which I put it down to the amount of exercise I do and the routine I like to follow. Whenever possible I like to get to bed early and I'm a good riser. That probably comes from my mum waking me and forcing me to get up when I was young and then, when I was older, having to open the gym early in the morning. I love my sleep and only ever have problems in the last couple of weeks of a diet, when I can get really hungry.

Prolonged periods of sleep are essential. This is the time when muscle repair and the release of essential hormones, which are essential for our bodies to continue to function, take place. There are also long-term benefits: good sleeping habits have been proven to prevent excess weight gain, heart disease and other potential health issues.

When you're asleep, the brain also takes the opportunity to detoxify (flush out unwanted cells), recharge and reorganise while you are sleeping. It firms up our memories and smoothes out the way we process information. This is why you feel so alert after a good night's sleep and are able to focus, concentrate and perform better whether at work or in exercise.

How much sleep you need varies from person to person, but falls somewhere between six and ten hours. Teenagers will be at the upper end of this scale, because they need sleep for their growth and development, and at the lower end, while there is no proof that older people need less sleep, research has shown that it becomes more difficult to sleep for an extended period of time once you pass the age of 60.

It's easy to say all this, but I know that some people don't find it easy to get to or stay asleep. Physical discomfort, anxiety, a brain still wide awake or just an unexplainable inability to get to sleep affects many people. It can be difficult, but there are ways in which you can give yourself the best chance possible, so I've rounded them up here.

Sweet dreams

Have a regular sleep pattern: Our bodies have a fantastic inner clock and respond to routine. Whenever possible, go to sleep in the evening, and get up and get active in the morning at the same times every day.

Create a bedtime routine: This doesn't mean just washing, cleaning your teeth and changing into clean pyjamas, but having a process of winding down that includes turning your screens off well before bedtime and creating a stress-free space in which you can write a diary, plan for the next day or read.

Prepare your sleep station: Make your sleeping area as comfortable as you can. Deal with the things that might bother you: tidy the room; make sure the curtains are fully closed; turn off computers, phones or rechargers or put them where you can't see their lights. Make the bed itself snug with pillows and covers that make you feel relaxed.

Watch what you eat and drink: Give your body a few hours to digest your evening meal before going to bed. However, don't go to bed hungry. Have a small snack like a cracker, some popcorn or a small bowl of cereal. It's also a good idea to avoid having tea, coffee or other drinks with caffeine after mid-afternoon, as the body can take five hours before its brain-stimulating effect wears off.

Exercise: Although science can't yet explain exactly why this is, research has shown that 30 minutes or more of moderate exercise during the day can aid sleep. One note of caution, though: exercising two hours or less before bedtime can have the reverse effect because the endorphins that released by exercise cause an increase in brain activity. So don't leave it too late to do that class or workout.

AFTER *LOVE ISLAND*

Leaving the villa was weird. I'd been in that bubble for 58 days. Back home there'd been a heatwave, and Theresa May had resigned and Boris Johnson had taken over as Prime Minister. World War III could have broken out and we wouldn't have known about it. In that last week the villa had begun to feel like a posh prison and, although I was gutted to be leaving, I wasn't going to dwell on it. *It is what it is, I thought. Time to make the best of it.*

You leave the same way you enter, back into that same room where the same producers check you're OK and then you're whisked off to the casting villa. I did *After Sun* and the *This Morning* interview with Eamonn Holmes and Ruth Langsford – and they still hadn't given me my phone back! You don't get much in the way of souvenirs either. They let you keep your case and I managed to smuggle out a few mementoes, including the *Love Island* branded washbag, toothbrush and condom packet (still sealed!). I'd also asked for a new water bottle while I was there and kept it under my bed to take home, but stupidly I put it down at the airport when someone asked for a photo and I lost it.

I finally got my phone back just before I got on the plane to fly home. By now, of course, I had some idea of how people had reacted to my time on the show, but I was still overwhelmed by the sheer numbers. When I got back to London, I headed straight to the ITV studios to watch the final, marvelling as my Instagram followers ticked up. I hit 1 million as I entered the building and it kept rising, finally peaking at 1.4 million.

Everyone wants a piece of you, particularly the press, and the first thing I needed was a management company. I wasn't under contract with Bold, the company I had been dealing with, as we'd agreed to see how things panned out on the show. Although there were now plenty of companies looking to sign me, I felt I owed Bold some loyalty. They had created the opportunity for me to go on the show and had always treated me fairly. It was a good choice, as they helped me through the following incredible months.

I felt I was a well-balanced guy who was ready for the fame that came from being on the show, but honestly nothing can prepare you for the reaction. The first time I ventured into Glasgow after I got back, I went with a friend. I expected a few people would want photos, but certainly not enough to hold up the traffic. I was so wrong. As soon as I got out of the car, I was approached and by the time I looked round again there was a crowd. Within minutes I had 500 people surrounding me, and had to get back in the car and give up the idea of shopping.

I can't deny I was enjoying myself. I love meeting people and chatting, and everyone I met – girls and guys – only wanted to be friendly. I know some of the other guys on the show had to deal with some aggressive idiots, but that never happened to me. Best of all, I finally got to go the freshers' events at universities around the country – when all my friends went to uni, I was busy working and that was something I always felt I missed out on.

Over the next 90 days I attended 85 events. Across the UK, I made personal appearances at clubs, opened stores, turned on Christmas lights and even appeared at Truckfest! It was mad. I was getting paid silly money for an hour's work, just to have a good time. To cap it all, I got to meet Craig David – again! He had left a message on the reunion programme inviting me to his TS5 pool party in Ibiza. I didn't need asking twice. I had tickets in the VIP section, but it got better. Midway through the show, he called me down to the stage. I was buzzing. It was one of the greatest nights of my life, and it wouldn't have happened without *Love Island*.

My friends witnessed the whole crazy circus. They'd laugh, because they knew exactly what everyone would ask. 'What was such and such like?' 'Are you still in touch with them all?' 'Are you seeing Belle?'

The truth wasn't very exciting. The thing is life is different in the villa. The circumstances mean you make strong friendships and bond with people you might have little in common with in normal life. However, when you get back into the real world, there are so many distractions and calls on your time, as well as the fact that Islanders live so far from each other, it's difficult to maintain that emotional intensity.

I did stay in touch with Joe. He really was my best friend in the villa and I count him as a friend. The others – as much as I still like them all – have already drifted away. And Belle? To be honest, it was never really going to happen. She had her life in London and I was settled in Glasgow. In the whirlwind of commitments after the show ended, we found it almost impossible to find time to meet up. We still got along really well when we managed to find time to speak on the phone, but we both knew that a long-term relationship was ultimately not viable.

I never went on *Love Island* to chase fame, but that celebrity lifestyle was looking attractive. The thought of going back to rising at 5am to open the gym had certainly lost some of its appeal. Some previous Islanders had gone on to TV presenting roles or become influencers, and those routes certainly opened themselves up to me. I took up an offer from TikTok to do some videos for them. They were just little fun pieces, often laughing at myself. I re-enacted the coupling scene with Anna (playing both parts) and did an over-the-top Craig David fanboy video, and I soon had 100,000 young followers – exactly the audience I was looking for. The press slated me for the videos: they didn't get TikTok at that point, and said they were immature and embarrassing. Instead of trusting my own instincts, I felt shamed into stopping doing them, which is something I regret now.

Fame is like a mist that descends and stops you seeing beyond your own nose. The adoration from complete strangers, the luxury lifestyle, the ridiculous sums you get for doing virtually nothing – it can all suck you into thinking someone you are not. I confess I lost myself for a short time. Letting those TikTok criticisms get to me was an example of that. It just wasn't like me. Under the pressure of celebrity in those months after *Love Island,* I felt the insecurities which I had when I was a young teenager returning.

It's difficult to explain the comedown from the highest of highs – experiencing the buzz of being on the show and the excitement of sudden fame – to the lowest of lows afterwards as you return to your life. I believe the producers did their very best to look after us, but whether it's the emptiness you feel, the weight of so many vicious social media posts or the freely available drink at endless parties, it can be a difficult time. Although the producers of the series do try to prepare you for this, there have been tragic consequences; Sophie Gradon and Mike Thalassitis both took their own lives after being on the show.

As 2020 approached I took stock and managed to catch myself, perhaps just in time. I had never been one for alcohol, but I was drinking more than I ever had. It wasn't a problem, I wasn't drinking more than a normal lad my age, but to me it was a sign I was letting myself go. I vowed to stop drinking and to diet. I usually have an iron will about these things, so the fact that I postponed it until the New Year so I could have fun at an Antony Joshua VIP party showed how much I had taken to the good life.

There's nothing like your mum telling you, 'You aren't a celebrity in this house' to bring you back to earth: I wasn't a superstar, I had been on TV once. What I did was run a fitness company and I did it pretty well. It was time to get back to what I did best. On Boxing Day my new fitness app was launched. It was the first time I had gone into a business partnership and I quickly regretted it. I had my own views on how and what the app should do, and it was frustrating to have such little control. I had recently turned down a potentially lucrative deal with the world's biggest fast food company as I was determined not to sell myself short on my principles. If I was going to do an app, I'd do it my way and so I pulled out of that project.

Those six months of madness had changed everything and there were times when my life was getting out of control. I have no regrets though. Some of my co-islanders have told me they wish they had never gone on *Love Island*, but it was honestly the best thing I ever did. Not only did I have the time of my life in the villa, but the TV exposure has helped me to do what I believe I am destined to do: make a difference.

What's important

If you want to live your best life, you need a number of elements to be in place – good relationships with friends and family, your health, a sensible work-life balance and the ability to enjoy your own company.

44. Know who your friends are

Good friends are invaluable. They can provide support, boost your self-esteem, have a massive impact on your general happiness and help connect you to your community and the world.

As an only child who is close to their parents and who has been in long-term relationships since they were a teenager, I still understand that I need my friends. They're not bound by family loyalties or expectations or by romantic ties, but they still care. They can appreciate your successes, support you in bad times and give you honest feedback on your actions, because they have a different viewpoint on your life. And it works two ways. By interacting with them and giving them support and encouragement in turn, you're picking up valuable life skills – and being a good person, of course!

Old friends, new friends

I've always found it pretty easy to make friends. As people saw on *Love Island*, I'm always looking to see the best in people, and my positive and eager-to-please attitude means they are usually happy to get to know me. I think I got along with all the Islanders, even in such an intense atmosphere, and I made some good friends in my chaperone, Sam, and Coco, one of the producers on the show. Of course, there are friends and then there are close friends.

I have a small group of close friends I trust implicitly – one of them is even my ex's brother! I'm comfortable with them and we have great fun together, especially on our trips to Ibiza, but I know we're there for each other at other times too. They have stood by me through all the ups and downs of recent years and I value their opinion. They have given me great support in helping me date again after *Love Island* and help me build my business.

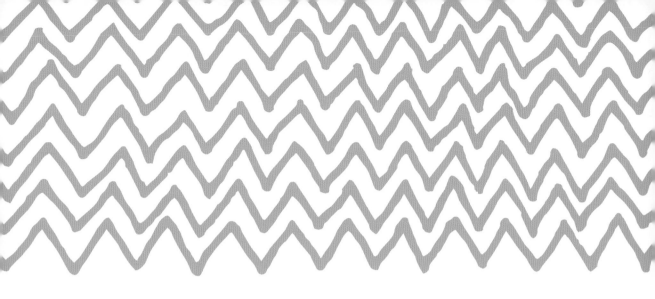

Boys and girls

My best mates are all guys, perhaps because I've always been in long-term relationships, but I believe it's equally possible to have girls as close friends. I have always got on well with girls and many who watched *Love Island* believed my lack of romantic success was due to the fact that the girls saw me as a friend not a prospective lover. I've also counted people older than me as friends. As an only child I'm used to talking to my parents and their friends, and as a trainer I got to know many older folk and valued the different perspective they had on life.

I've also lost friends over the years. It happens. A change of circumstances, some kind of crisis or just a drifting apart can all end a friendship you might have thought was going to last forever. Coming out of *Love Island* was an important moment for me, because I discovered who wanted to be friends with me for who I was and who just wanted a bit of reflected fame. My grandmother used to say: 'Life is like a bus, people get on and get off.' I always try to see the good in people, but if I can't trust them or they're not good for me to be around, I'm happy to let them go. When I'm done, I'm done. There's no going back.

45. Make your parents proud

We often take the relationship with our parents for granted. Sometimes they can seem too strict, like they lack understanding or even appear not to care. But if you nurture the bond with your mum and dad, there's so much to gain.

My mum's the best friend I have. Anyone who spends any time with me gets to realise that pretty quickly. We live within minutes of each other, work together on various projects and she shares my positive outlook on life. I tell her everything (and I mean everything) and she gives me advice on every aspect of my life. Some of it – such as opinions on some of my friends – have caused rows, but she's always proved right in the end! I have a different relationship with my dad. We're close too, but he's calmer and more reserved, and we have a more traditional relationship. We've always been a close family and I believe that's the bedrock which has enabled me to become the man I am.

Appreciate what they do

I haven't always been the perfect son, but as I've grown up, I've learned to appreciate what they've done and continue to do for me. Of course, we argue, sometimes heatedly, but we do so in the knowledge that we love and need each other, and with a little space and time we will resolve our differences. My parents have sacrificed so much for me and have given me unconditional love, despite not always receiving it back! I also know that I'm privileged and, for a host of different reasons, not everybody is lucky enough to have parents who are around or parents who do that. If you can, though, there is so much to be gained from having a strong relationship with your parents, because they can be counsellors, careers advisors, companions and even friends – and they do it all just for love.

It's not always easy. They can seem dictatorial, hypocritical, unfair, old-fashioned or have a view on your life that seems so far from the reality of it. The truth is that you probably won't change their outlook. You can, however, work on your own flaws to try to make the relationship work better. If you succeed, you'll be the one who benefits.

How to have a great relationship with your mum and dad

Talk to them: These are the people who know you best and genuinely care about you, so keep the lines of communication open, even if you're not getting along. Stay in touch, whether you're living in the same house or miles away from home. When I go on holiday, I always talk to my mum every day on the phone. Letting her share my thoughts and emotions just strengthens the bond between us.

Be honest: If you want your parents' support and help, they need to understand you. That means telling them the truth and including them in your life. Talk to them when things go wrong, as well as about your successes and dreams. Let them meet your friends and anyone important in your life, and make sure they know what you want out of life.

Be grateful: Most parents will do anything for their kids, so the very least you can do is show some gratitude. Accept them for what they are and what they can offer. I get my 'reach for the stars' mentality from my mum and she still helps me believe I can do anything and be anyone I want to be. My dad has a more measured and cautious view on life and, although I listen, I don't pay too much heed to what he says about my future plans. On the other hand, if he gives me advice on fixing my car or putting up shelves, I'm all ears.

Respect their opinions: The accepted ways of doing things change so fast in modern life. It can be difficult for some people, especially if they're set in their ways, to keep up. Your parents might not share all your values, standards of behaviour, choice in clothes etc, but remember it was probably the same with their parents when they were young. On the other hand, they have life experience and know you better than most, so even if you don't agree, give them the respect they deserve.

Parents are people too: While they've always been your mum and dad and act like you're the only thing in their lives that matters, it's sometimes easy to forget that they have a life away from you. As much as they might hide it, parents have relationship stresses, work issues, times they feel down too. Take time to treat them as you would a best friend – give them space, try to understand their moods, talk to them and, if you can, do something to help them.

Cherish your time together: It can be a difficult fact to face, but your parents will almost certainly pass away before you and leave you with only the memories. Do your best to make sure those memories are good ones. Enjoy the time you spend together, make sure you know them as people and make sure they know how much you love them – before it's too late.

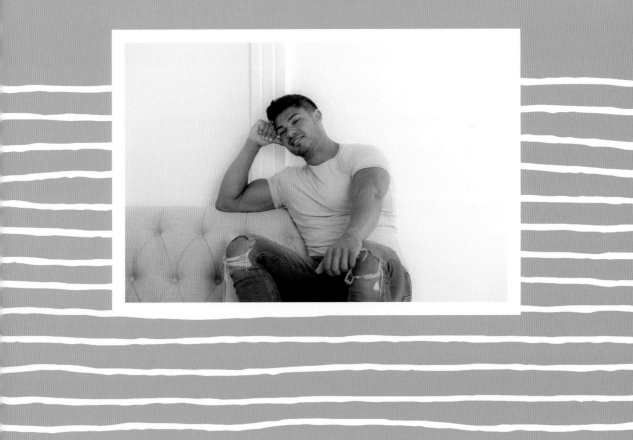

46. Time alone

Being alone is definitely not the same as being lonely. Spending time with other people is vital for our wellbeing, but so too is spending time on our own.

As an only child, being alone has always seemed a perfectly natural state for me, although I'm aware that not everyone feels the same. Some like the buzz of conversation and the comfort of having other people around all the time, but I've always needed to spend some time on my own and I would recommend it to anyone.

The key to enjoying being by yourself is inner contentment. You have to like yourself – and if you don't, you need to ask yourself what needs to change. When it comes to your own character, you might take other people's views on board, but your opinion is the only one that really matters. After all, if you don't like your own company, how can you expect others to like it? Outside influences can often be the most negative, though, and even when you're alone they're just a DM or a call away. Use time on your own to unplug and switch off from technology completely.

Make the most of that me time

Treat that time on your own as a luxury, not some kind of purgatory you have to endure while you wait for friends to turn up or it's time to go out. We spend so much of our lives compromising, being selfless and looking out for others, but this is an opportunity to focus on you – so take it. It can be a valuable chance to assess and refocus your life, to escape stress, recharge your batteries and enjoy doing exactly what you want, whether it's baking a cake, watching a film or reading.

There are some things you might choose to do alone. It is not rude or anti-social and you don't have to feel guilty about it. Next time you're out with friends, take a look at the number of people who are doing the same thing on their own. It's not unusual and definitely not weird to go for a walk or see a movie alone. Personally, I like to train alone. I've never enjoyed having a training partner. I like to go into my own world, focus on what I want to achieve and not be distracted by others.

When they're always there, it's so easy to take our friends and family for granted. If you have time away from them, you might find yourself missing them and noticing what's great about being with them. Understanding what you appreciate in them will make your time together even better.

47. Work-life balance

For me, the perfect work-life balance is something of a myth, because work and life aren't separate, and if you adopt a more flexible approach to how you use your time it will help you achieve your goals.

Google 'work-life balance', and you'll find millions of articles and thousands of books exploring the subject, and giving guidance on how to get it right. A lot of it is sensible advice on switching off, and making time for yourself and those you love. Personally, though, I find it hard to separate work from life. Work is – and has been since I started out – an inextricable part of my life.

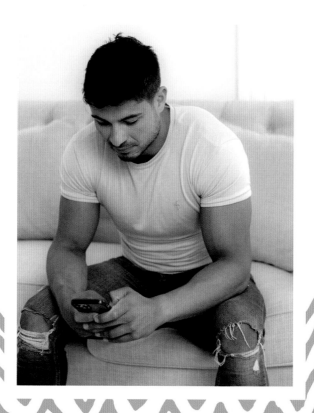

For many years I worked like anything to get my gym business off the ground. For a long time, it was pretty much all I did and I struggled to find time for my girlfriend and my family, let alone myself. When I complained, my mum would tell me it would all be worth it in the end and she often quoted one of her favourite phrases: 'Later is greater!' She was right – it was what I wanted to do. I was driven, and making a success of the gym was more important to me than partying with friends or lounging on the sofa watching Netflix.

How do you break it down?

As I see it, the ideal formula isn't necessarily eight hours' work plus eight hours' play plus eight hours' sleep. For me it's more flexible than that. The real balance for a perfect life is in how you go about what makes you feel happy and fulfilled. Understand what you value in life, what you're seeking to achieve and how you plan to get there. It might be to progress your career, to spend as much time with particular people as possible, to follow a passion such as sport or art, or to dedicate your time to helping others.

The balance you arrive at depends on how you choose to reach those goals, and the right balance for you is the one that helps you succeed. This will inevitably involve some sacrifice, whether it's financial, social or giving up certain activities, even if it's only for a while, but if there is a golden equation in which you can have everything at once, I've yet to see it.

Goals and flexibility

My goals are what inspire me to work hard. When I was younger the goal was establishing the gym and now it's about taking my fitness message to a mass audience. They both took my time and focus. But the balance can change. When I came out of *Love Island*, my focus changed for a while to having fun. I was able to hang out with my friends and catch up on 'lost time'. After a few months, I chose to return to a 'work first' mentality, because that was what I wanted to prioritise. I changed the equation. I dare say I will change again as I get older and my ambitions will change.

48. A strong sense of self

If you're going to live a happy life, it's essential to discover who you are and to actively like that person, but it's also important to realise that we can all be different people at different times and that you can always improve on who you are.

I'm 25 now. I've been a few different versions of me in the short time I've been alive. I was a cheerful little lad, an insecure teenager, a young man with a bit of a swagger and plenty of other incarnations in between. I recognise all those people as me, but I don't feel that any of them are who I am now.

We all change, especially in the years from 11 to 21, and some of us carry on changing for a long time after that. I've grown up and learned more about myself and the world. I've also had experiences which have had an effect on me: romantic relationships that have left me feeling either euphoric, devastated or guilty; business plans that have come to fruition or that haven't worked out in the way I hoped they would; and people I've met who have inspired me or let me down. And then there was the intense experience of *Love Island* with its massive highs and gut-wrenching lows.

Find out how you fit in

We all grow and change as we learn more fully how we fit in with the world. I feel I know myself quite well now. I have a positive attitude to life; I care deeply about those close to me; I want to make a difference to people; I want to think the best of everyone; I have high expectations of other people's behaviour; I put effort into my appearance; and I work hard. I also know what I want, dream big and believe I can accomplish great things.

Understanding who you are and what you're about isn't easy, but it's central to your self-esteem and happiness. It takes in not only your external persona – how you present yourself to the world and interact with people – but also your internal character, which determines what you value and what you want to be. And, if you're not happy about what you see or just want to be better, then all of those things are open to change any time you choose. Assessing your own personal identity is all about questioning yourself. Here are a few questions that I sometimes ask myself and which might start you thinking:

Who do you think you are?

▶ What aspect of myself makes me most proud?

▶ What is my biggest achievement in life?

▶ What experiences have helped forge who I am and which have I ignored?

▶ What disappointment or painful experience did I get through and how did I do it?

▶ What qualities do I appreciate in others, but lack in myself?

▶ What values do I believe in, but don't live up to?

▶ Who am I trying to impress – my family, my friends, myself or nobody?

▶ What would I think if I met myself?

49. Staying healthy

Health and fitness simply can't be a short-term goal. There's no way round it – if you want to enjoy life to the full in the future, you will need to commit to looking after your body now and in the years ahead.

Here's what would happen when I was a trainer, not just once, but over and over. I'd work with someone to help them reach their fitness and weight goals. At that point they'd say, 'Thanks for your help, Anton. I think I can take it from here.' Fair enough. They were paying me good money and it wasn't going to go on forever. I could tell, though, which ones would be back in maybe six months or a year having put the weight back on – and invariably I was right. Staying fit and healthy isn't something that can be ticked off and then put aside. It just doesn't work like that.

Just as you might regularly check your bank balance or the oil levels in the car, so you need to be aware of your physical health. You have to try understand how you're feeling and decide what alterations to your lifestyle – such as your diet, exercise, alcohol intake or social activities – you might need to make. It's your body and your responsibility. No one else can do it for you.

Learn to enjoy exercise

Exercise needs to be part of your life, as much as working, eating and sleeping, so you will need to have an enthusiasm for it. I believe exercise should a source of enjoyment, never a chore, and I always look forward to my daily workout. I enjoy the whole process, the focus, the exertion and the feeling when I finish. If I miss a day due to other commitments, I don't feel guilty, just a little empty, as if I'd missed an episode of my favourite TV show or a football match.

There's no shame in not liking running or swimming or even going to the gym, but from the hundreds of forms of exercise available find something you enjoy – and something else to move onto if you get bored of that. As I've said, I've taken up boxing training. It's given me a buzz that I was maybe missing in my gym and cardio work, and it's the last thing I want to cross out of my diary.

Eat it and sleep it

Diet is the second pillar of a healthy life. We all have a good idea of how much and what we should be eating and drinking, but it's all too easy to put that knowledge aside amid all the pressures of our lives. The importance of what we eat can't be stressed enough. A diet is not a short-term weight-loss programme but a life-long understanding of how we can give our body what it requires for healthy living.

Rest and relaxation are just as essential to your long-term health. Stress and anxiety can do physical harm and you should do all you can to deal with the causes and relieve the symptoms. The benefits of getting the required hours of quality sleep have been covered elsewhere in this book, but switching off and unwinding with some quiet time, spending time with friends and loved ones (the human touch – a massage or even just a hug – is proven to reduce blood pressure) and laughter, which is a great source of relaxation, also make a significant contribution to your health.

I know I've talked about these a lot, but it really does all come down to exercise, diet and rest. Get those right – and keep them up – and you'll be set.

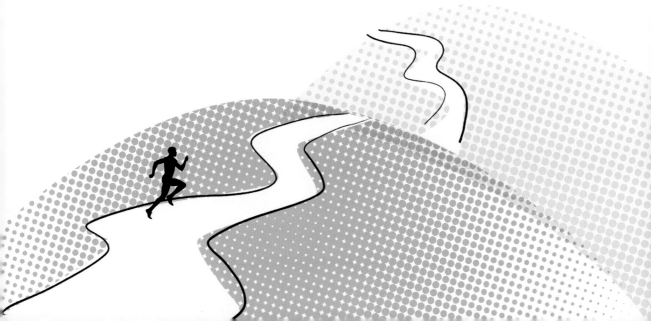

50. Live your best life

Life involves goals, challenges, triumphs and setbacks. Our best chance of success is to find an energy that supports our aspirations and sees us through our struggles.

You are the author of your own story. Life isn't something that just happens to you, it's what you choose to make of it. That comes from doing something, heading in a direction, having a goal – no matter how small. Taking control of your life means admitting that there are no excuses, only choices. Sure, there are going to be obstacles along the way, but they only go to prove you're moving forward. Whether we achieve or are disappointed, we have to get up and go again, re-evaluate our goals and our plans, and never stop trying.

Components for success

Throughout this book, I have talked about the importance of setting personal goals in your life. However small they are, these are your milestones towards living your best life. The secret to successfully achieving them is to be committed and to work hard – and resilience and sheer determination, particularly in the face of adversity, will get you quite a long way.

In the short term, working to meet a deadline, grinding through the last two weeks of calorie-cutting or pounding the streets as you train for a marathon, can be punishing, but ultimately rewarding – reaching that goal will make it all worthwhile. However, unless you have super human powers of application and endurance, sustaining efforts that you find uninspiring, inconvenient or too draining will be impossible. Always keep in mind that the long-term motivation to keep working towards your personal goals depends on your enjoyment of the process.

Energy sources

Keeping a constant level of energy is the secret to making the best possible things happen. Much of this book has pointed you towards the ways in which you can continue to source this energy. Your physical health – starting with self-care and basic fitness – is paramount. Increasing your exercise programme will increase your fitness levels and your energy. You shouldn't fear over-exercise, as your body will produce more energy to meet your needs. Being strong, flexible and responsive will prepare you for most physical challenges you will face in life.

Your diet also has a direct impact on your day-to-day energy levels. An over-reliance on high-calorie, low-nutrient foods will not fully sustain your everyday tasks and will lead to you putting on weight. Even if you're happy with your weight, the proportions of carbs, protein and fats you consume can significantly affect your blood sugar levels. In an earlier chapter I wrote how our carb-based and low-fat obsession can create a rollercoaster effect. My experience is that a stronger reliance on protein and fats can help stabilise your mood throughout the day.

Let your passion motivate you

Physical fitness and your diet can affect brain activity and mental sharpness too. This is important because your internal drive is vital in maintaining your desire to make changes in your life. The confidence, positivity, visualisation and a focus on desired outcomes that I discussed earlier can all be used to create long-term motivation.

Finally, there is no substitute for a genuine passion for what you're trying to achieve. Find something you love doing, and you'll always give it 100%. If we can approach the key experiences of life – our work, relationships and pursuits – with enthusiasm, our chances of success are so much greater.

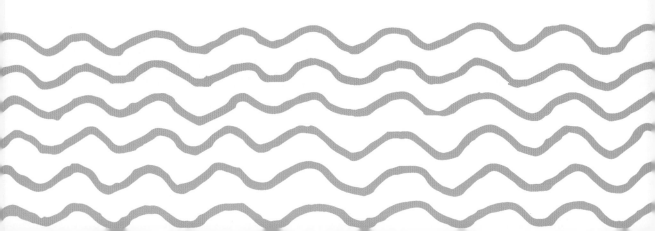

LOOKING TO THE FUTURE

In September 2019, I was chosen to be an Ambassador for World Merit working on their youth movement in conjunction with the UN's Sustainable Development programme. It was an honour and an unbelievable opportunity. In the first few months of 2020, before lockdown, I toured schools promoting health and wellbeing. The celebrity factor paid off; the kids now knew who I was and were willing to engage with what I had to say. Their reaction gave me so much confidence and reassured me that I was on the right road. I had dreamed of being able to impact lives in a positive way and at last it was happening. I truly felt my whole life had been leading up to doing this.

My main focus now is an app and fitness mat I have been developing. The mat consists of 12 coloured squares and the app takes users through a series of low-impact combinations of feet and arm movements safely and effectively. I believe the app can help me reach thousands of children, and adults too, and instil the confidence in them to lead fit and healthy lives. If I can use my celebrity profile to launch the project into the stratosphere, it will be both the culmination of a plan made some years ago and a dream come true.

I don't have to look far for inspiration.

The famous US trainer Shaun T is a big inspiration to me. His Beachbody, Insanity and Hip Hop Abs products have sold millions and have shown how easily you can follow a fitness and muscle-building programme at home. The way Shaun connects with people through fitness, his motivational power, his positivity and his desire to help people feel better about themselves is incredible. I am still learning so much from him.

I have so many great hopes for my fitness project and I hope it will be a success. That doesn't stop me having other dreams and schemes, though. I've always enjoyed doing TV work and given the right opportunity would love to be back on the screen. I still get offers for reality and dating shows and, while the financial rewards are great and it can be fun, what I would really LOVE is to present a fitness-related TV show along the lines of Netflix's *Strong* or the US series *The Biggest Loser*. One day I'd also love to appear on the front cover of *Men's Health* magazine. That would be the recognition that I had successfully transformed from a reality star to a respected fitness personality.

I TRULY FELT MY WHOLE LIFE HAD BEEN LEADING UP TO DOING THIS.

My mum, and my dad, once envisaged me working with them in the family popcorn business. I wanted to find my own way and show I could make it on my own. Now, having done that, I feel ready to take over the company when they no longer feel able or want to run it. They've worked so hard over the years that no one could begrudge them putting their feet up. They've always been happy to operate it without many changes and have done so very successfully, but I already find myself formulating plans to expand the business. I have a keen entrepreneurial sense and feel I could link the healthy qualities of popcorn with the wider fitness message.

Maybe by that time I'll have a family too. I have so much to achieve in the months and years immediately ahead, I haven't really had time to consider a serious relationship. If it comes along so be it, but I can wait. To repeat my mum's classic line, 'Later will be greater.'

THANK YOU!

Writing this book has been such a rewarding experience for me, and expressing the ideas, values and actions that I believe can help all of us has allowed me to focus my own thoughts about how I live my life as well. In the course of writing the book, I have changed my diet, begun and ended a new relationship, and initiated several exciting new projects, and I hope that reading this helps you make lots of good things happen in your lives too.

I believe that we can make our own success and happiness, but I also understand the importance of the support of those who love us. Evaluating what has made me the person I am has made me realise how lucky I have been to have the love of my family every step of the way. They have made the journey so much easier, and I will be forever grateful.

And, of course, I also want to thank all my wonderful fans, because every single one of you is very much part of my achievements, and I wouldn't be doing what I am now if you hadn't liked me and responded to me. You're fantastic and I'm very lucky to have your support.

Anton

@Anton_Danyluk

Anton Danyluk

@AntonDanyluk

@Anton_Danyluk

Anton Danyluk